Re

Dr Tom Smith has been writing since 1977, after spen... six years in general practice and seven years in medical research. He writes the 'Doctor, Doctor' column in *The Guardian* on Saturdays, and has written three humorous books, *Doctor, Have You Got a Minute?*, *A Seaside Practice* and *Going Loco*, all published by Short Books. His other books for Sheldon Press include *Heart Attacks: Prevent and Survive*, *Living with Alzheimer's Disease*, *Overcoming Back Pain*, *Coping with Bowel Cancer*, *Coping with Heartburn and Reflux*, *Coping with Age-related Memory Loss*, *101 Questions to Ask Your Doctor*, *How to Get the Best from Your Doctor*, *Coping with Kidney Disease*, *Osteoporosis: Prevent and Treat* and *Coping Successfully with Prostate Cancer*.

Overcoming Common Problems Series

Selected titles

A full list of titles is available from Sheldon Press,
36 Causton Street, London SW1P 4ST and on our website at
www.sheldonpress.co.uk

101 Questions to Ask Your Doctor
Dr Tom Smith

Asperger Syndrome in Adults
Dr Ruth Searle

The Assertiveness Handbook
Mary Hartley

Assertiveness: Step by step
Dr Windy Dryden and Daniel Constantinou

Backache: What you need to know
Dr David Delvin

Body Language: What you need to know
David Cohen

Bulimia, Binge-eating and their Treatment
Professor J. Hubert Lacey, Dr Bryony Bamford
and Amy Brown

The Cancer Survivor's Handbook
Dr Terry Priestman

The Chronic Pain Diet Book
Neville Shone

Cider Vinegar
Margaret Hills

Coeliac Disease: What you need to know
Alex Gazzola

Confidence Works
Gladeana McMahon

Coping Successfully with Pain
Neville Shone

Coping Successfully with Prostate Cancer
Dr Tom Smith

Coping Successfully with Psoriasis
Christine Craggs-Hinton

Coping Successfully with Ulcerative Colitis
Peter Cartwright

Coping Successfully with Varicose Veins
Christine Craggs-Hinton

Coping Successfully with Your Hiatus Hernia
Dr Tom Smith

Coping Successfully with Your Irritable Bowel
Rosemary Nicol

Coping When Your Child Has Cerebral Palsy
Jill Eckersley

Coping with Age-related Memory Loss
Dr Tom Smith

Coping with Birth Trauma and Postnatal Depression
Lucy Jolin

Coping with Bowel Cancer
Dr Tom Smith

Coping with Bronchitis and Emphysema
Dr Tom Smith

Coping with Candida
Shirley Trickett

Coping with Chemotherapy
Dr Terry Priestman

Coping with Chronic Fatigue
Trudie Chalder

Coping with Coeliac Disease
Karen Brody

Coping with Compulsive Eating
Dr Ruth Searle

Coping with Diabetes in Childhood and Adolescence
Dr Philippa Kaye

Coping with Diverticulitis
Peter Cartwright

Coping with Dyspraxia
Jill Eckersley

Coping with Early-onset Dementia
Jill Eckersley

Coping with Eating Disorders and Body Image
Christine Craggs-Hinton

Coping with Envy
Dr Windy Dryden

Coping with Epilepsy in Children and Young People
Susan Elliot-Wright

Coping with Family Stress
Dr Peter Cheevers

Coping with Gout
Christine Craggs-Hinton

Coping with Hay Fever
Christine Craggs-Hinton

Coping with Headaches and Migraine
Alison Frith

Coping with Hearing Loss
Christine Craggs-Hinton

Overcoming Common Problems Series

Overcoming Common Problems Series

Overcoming Common Problems

Reducing Your Risk of Dementia

DR TOM SMITH

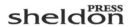

First published in Great Britain in 2011

Sheldon Press
36 Causton Street
London SW1P 4ST
www.sheldonpress.co.uk

British Library Cataloguing-in-Publication Data
A catalogue record for this book is available from the British Library

ISBN 978–1–84709–146–8
eBook ISBN 978–1–84709–219–9

1 3 5 7 9 10 8 6 4 2

Typeset by Kenneth Burnley Studios, Wirral, Cheshire
Printed in Great Britain by Ashford Colour Press

Produced on paper from sustainable forests

For my late parents,
Tom and Jeannie Smith, of Glasgow then Lincoln,
who spent their lives in the service of the
handicapped and underprivileged.
They expected little out of life,
but gave so much love to so many,
and especially to me

Contents

Introduction

The greatest health news story in September 2010, splashed all over the national press and featuring as the first story in the television news, was that if we all took lashings of vitamin B we would not develop dementia. We were told that a new study had proven almost beyond doubt that this very cheap medication, not even a drug – a vitamin, no less – would save billions in health care costs. It would cut to almost zero the numbers (the tabloids estimated them in millions) of us who would otherwise face our last years in care homes. It would let us enjoy our seventies, eighties and even nineties in good mental health, alert and happy. And best of all we would not be a burden on our families and carers. The future would be a utopia, in which old age would be transformed into the best years of our lives.

It sounds wonderful. Yet even on the first day of such brilliant news, a few newspapers tossed in a few doubts. *The Guardian*, I'm pleased to say (I write a column in its Saturday magazine), was one of them. After reporting the good news, it finished with the not-so-good. The Alzheimer's Society, my colleague wrote, warned that it had already conducted trials using vitamin B, and found that it had failed to make a difference to the prevention or the treatment of dementia.

Sadly, that's a pattern of breaking news that family doctors like me have had to bear for many years. News of any 'breakthrough' is often greeted with headlines, articles and news stories that don't fully reflect the content of the research findings. Progressive diseases like dementia and multiple sclerosis, for which we don't yet have satisfactory remedies, are particularly subject to reports like this, boosting hopes but eventually letting people down. And when it eventually dawns on people that the 'cure-all' doesn't actually do what has been promised, the newspapers aren't there to apologize or even to mention the bad news.

So I'm afraid that this book isn't sensational. It won't promise a cure or methods of perfect prevention of dementia. It does, however, bring together what is known about the causes of dementia and how each of us can do our best to prevent ourselves developing it early or, hopefully, at all. Medicine isn't an exact science. Some of us are programmed from early in life to be at higher risk than others from dementia as we age. The best we can do, if we are in that group, is to try to postpone its onset. On the other hand, the vast majority of us may avoid dementia altogether if we follow sensible guidelines.

My aim in writing *Reducing Your Risk of Dementia* is to explain why we should heed the guidelines, and what we, as individuals, can do to maximize our own chances of keeping a healthy brain into a happy and, hopefully, healthy old age.

Why do we need an individual approach to dementia prevention? Because there is no enthusiasm among the health authorities to initiate a prevention programme for the general public – unlike those for, say, breast cancer and prostate cancer. An editorial in the *British Medical Journal* (*BMJ*) of 14 August 2010 posed the question 'Can dementia be prevented?' Its answer was 'Modifiable risk factors exist but targeted public health programmes are not warranted.'

That's disappointing for us all, but reasonable. I'll explain why the *BMJ* came to this conclusion later, but it doesn't exclude general practitioners (GPs) like me from trying to help. So this book will describe all the 'modifiable risk factors' to which the editorial refers, and look at how we, as individuals, can change them to our probable advantage. It is, after all, up to us to do what we can to help ourselves, as the lifestyle and behaviour that raise the risk of dementia are under our own control, not our doctor's or our medical team's. Sadly, nothing in medicine is infallible: despite making the appropriate changes in our lives, we may still develop dementia. The good news, however, is that if we do our best we will almost certainly delay its onset and slow its progress. Putting off dementia for ten years or so is a benefit, even if it eventually catches up with us.

Dementia is not a single illness, which is why this book is not entitled *Reducing Your Risk of Alzheimer's Disease*. Essentially it has two components: loss of memory and loss of intellect. The two are not the same. Their causes can range from multiple small strokes to primary brain cell disease, and their prevention needs different approaches. The book starts, therefore, by describing the types of dementia and what we know about their causes. How common dementia is, how early it can start, how easily the early stages can be missed, and how long we can manage to live with it, are all dealt with in the next chapters. Each chapter from then onwards takes one 'risk factor' in turn, and explains its link with dementia and how we can minimize our personal risk from it.

In August 2010 Dr Elizabeth England of Birmingham University wrote a definitive thesis about the survival of people in the UK after they have been diagnosed with dementia. I wholly agree with her main message that everyone involved in its diagnosis and treatment needs better education and training. That goes for us, too, if we are at risk, have early dementia ourselves or are caring for someone with dementia. I have tried to answer Dr England's plea on behalf of us all.

1

Know your enemy – the dementias

If you wish to prevent yourself from developing dementia, it's best to know what you are up against and why it is so difficult to take definitive action against it. This chapter explains what dementia is and describes the different forms it takes. You may find it a bit depressing, but look upon it as a challenge to be defeated rather than as anything to be afraid of.

Probably the best, and most understandable, definition of dementia is that of the World Health Organization (WHO). To have dementia, people must

- have a decline in memory that impairs their ability to live normally;
- have difficulties in thinking and in processing of information, sufficient to disturb their normal ability to live with others in family life and work;
- have no clouding of consciousness, such as sleepiness;
- have emotional and behaviour changes that cause them to have social problems and to lack motivation;
- have had all these symptoms for at least six months.

You might think, from this comprehensive list, that if you do show all of these symptoms you must have dementia. It isn't so simple. For example, temporary problems with memory may be due to other causes. A minor stroke, epilepsy, abuse of drugs and alcohol, brain injuries and tumours, depression, an underactive thyroid gland ('myxoedema') and pernicious anaemia can all lead to these symptoms – and their effects are treatable and reversible. So it is incumbent on doctors, when dementia is suspected, to rule them out before settling on the diagnosis.

Some medicines – mainly sedatives, tranquillizers and anti-epilepsy drugs – and chronic poisoning with industrial and agricultural-chemicals such as lead and organophosphates (pesticides) will also produce the WHO list of symptoms. Then there are the long-term effects of drugs of abuse, such as cocaine and ecstasy, on the brains of regular users. The dementia-like symptoms produced by these chemicals are not so easy to reverse.

In 2000 I was asked to write *Living with Alzheimer's Disease*, a book for people looking after relatives and friends, and for people in the early stages of the illness. I started it with a letter from Jean, a 59-year-old schoolteacher:

> I have just been given the news that I have early Alzheimer's disease. I went to my doctor because I haven't been getting on well at school. I was forgetting things, being a bit muddled sometimes, and I thought it was just my age. But tests show that it is Alzheimer's. As you can imagine, I'm shocked beyond belief. What lies ahead of me? Will I be able to cope for at least a while? What can I do for myself to improve my outlook? Do I face a hopeless decline into senseless oblivion? Please be honest with me.

How did I reply? She had written to me because she had taught my daughter and wanted a second opinion, so I felt I had to take things further than just answer her query in my newspaper column. I felt I had to find out if she had had all the investigations to rule out reversible causes of her symptoms, so I wrote a very tactful letter to her doctor, who was a respected and friendly colleague I had known for years. It's difficult for doctors to do this, as we have to make sure we don't seem to be casting any doubt on a colleague's management of a case.

I needn't have worried. He was just as keen as I was to clarify her position. She had had a head injury (a car crash after which she had concussion for a day) two months before. Could her symptoms be the result of a clot on the brain surface caused by a subdural bleed? He had ruled that out. He had also ruled out thyroid underactivity, depression, pernicious anaemia and age-related memory loss. She had no headaches, blurred or double vision, or nerve problems that might indicate a brain tumour that could be removed. Examination of her eyes showed a normal retina, ruling out excess pressure inside the brain. Even with all these checks, her doctor was arranging a brain scan for her to make sure nothing was missed. Blood tests showed that she didn't have anaemia and that there was no evidence of chronic poisoning.

We were left with the original diagnosis.

Jean retired early and gave up driving her car. Her sister Alice came to live with her, and the two ladies faced the future together. They kept each other interested in their community and their interests, which varied from quilt-making to hill walking, the arts, music and history. For eight years Jean had a reasonably good life, before her dementia and Alice's physical frailty led her to enter a nursing home. In 2011, eleven years after that letter, she is in the final stages, largely in bed, not speaking, not knowing who or where she is, and under full-time nursing care. She is just 70.

Could she have prevented this too early descent into what for her was 'oblivion'? It is impossible to say. She never smoked and hardly drank alcohol. There was no family history of early dementia. The only incidents in her life that might have been related to it were two serious head injuries, both related to car crashes, one ten years before the onset of her symptoms, and the one we knew about in early 2000. Neither was her fault, so she could not have avoided them. We could probably find such incidents in the lives of most people of her age, so it isn't rational to blame them.

However, there is a bright side to this tragedy. Because her illness was identified early, Jean had eight genuinely happy years living with her sister and her friends. She kept up her interests, physical and mental, for as long as she could – longer, in fact, than I or her doctor would have predicted from our original assessment of the depth of her dementia. She set her mind to enjoying what she had left, and did so wonderfully well. I'm sure that this attitude helped to make her final years much more bearable, and perhaps even slowed the progress of her dementia.

I suppose the message from Jean is that, even when dementia is clouding our thoughts, memory and intellect, there is still hope that we can improve things for a while, and that the 'while' can last for some years, if we apply ourselves and enjoy our relationships with the people closest and dearest to us. It is a thought to keep hold of as we look to the future.

Types of dementia – Alzheimer's and the rest

Asked about types of dementia, most people will probably answer 'Alzheimer's disease' and struggle to name any others. A few will add 'mini-stroke disease', but stop there. So here is a short run-down of the illnesses we clump together as the 'dementias', of which Alzheimer's makes up around two-thirds of all cases and mini-stroke disease around a quarter. The other, much rarer types of dementia account for the remaining one in 12 cases.

Alzheimer's disease

In 1906, Dr Alois Alzheimer reported on the microscopic findings in the brain of a woman whom he considered to have a rare mental illness. Her first symptom had been unfounded and overwhelming jealousy, which was soon followed by loss of memory, difficulty in speaking, nervousness and inability to manage her household finances. She became paranoid, accusing the people around her of constantly talking in a disparaging way about her. She deteriorated quickly into complete dementia, and died within months.

Dr Alzheimer was meticulous in his attention to detail. He published pictures of the microscopic appearance of the dead woman's brain, in which he described two main differences from the normal brain. The first was that many of the neurofibrils – structures that normally extend from nerve cells, like the spreading branches of a tree, and that pass on the nerve messages from one cell to all the others around it – were tangled. They criss-crossed each other in a haphazard way so that they were no longer in direct contact with fibrils from the adjacent nerve cells. Dr Alzheimer assumed that this meant that the cells involved in tangles could not communicate with the rest of the brain.

The second finding was the presence of areas, called 'plaques', of a strange, smooth material with no visible internal structure between and around the brain cells, and taking up much of the space that cells had previously occupied. This substance we now know as 'amyloid'.

It became accepted that the combination of the tangles and the plaques was the definitive post-mortem sign of Alzheimer's disease.

The argument is still ongoing about whether the plaques cause or are the result of damage to brain cells. Does amyloid kill off the cells, leading to the disease, or is it a special scar tissue produced by the brain after the cells die off? The tangles are assumed to be a sign that the damaged but surviving brain cells are disorganized and cannot perform their function of passing on electrical or chemical messages between themselves. As they are almost always found together in the same areas of the brain, could the amyloid cause the tangles, or vice versa, or are both the result of an unknown inflammatory process, perhaps induced by a virus infection? If we could answer these questions we might be able to stop the process and even reverse it.

Where do we stand in 2011 on this subject? We know now that plaques and tangles are not exclusive to Alzheimer's disease. They occur in other brain disorders, such as Down's syndrome and Creutzfeldt-Jakob disease (CJD, the human form of 'mad cow disease' that so frightened the world in the late 1990s). Tangles and amyloid are even found, post-mortem, in a few people who have never had dementia in life.

An odd point to make is that what we now call Alzheimer's disease isn't really what Professor Alzheimer described. His patient's case is much more typical of CJD than of the usual pattern of the disease we now call after him. She progressed from apparent normality to death within a year or two. Alzheimer's usually takes much longer – sometimes as long as twenty years from first symptom to the final stages.

Naturally, researchers have concentrated on the relationship between these odd brain changes and the development of the illness. Teams of geneticists, biochemists, neurologists, microbiologists and brain-imaging specialists have been working together to try to identify the initial change in the brain that leads to them, and, most importantly of all, how to stop and perhaps reverse them.

These teams have been working for a long time. In the early 1990s I was privileged to be appointed as secretary to a group of professors of research institutes, all of whom were working on different aspects of the changes in the brain associated with Alzheimer's disease. Their ultimate aim was to find medicines to combat it. They saw promise in several biochemical pathways that might keep affected brain cells functioning and prevent the formation of amyloid. I can't believe that it was nearly twenty years ago, and that we still don't have anything that makes more than a minor difference to the disease. In 2011, the light at the end of the tunnel is getting brighter, but reaching it is still years away.

One promising route towards preventing dementia, which occupied much of my professorial colleagues' time, was the brain transmitter acetylcholine. It was known to help the transmission of messages between brain cells: the more acetylcholine we could amass in the tissues between our brain cells, the theory went, the more active and effective the cells were, and the less likely they were to succumb to degeneration and inactivity. Years of research were spent in trials of a drug that was known to stop the breakdown of acetylcholine in the brain, only to find that its probable adverse effects might be worse than its benefits. That line of research was finally given up, with great sadness because the initial trials had shown so much promise.

I was heartened, therefore, to read in December 2010 that the acetylcholine story has been revived. Dr Jack Mellor of Bristol University's School of Physiology and Pharmacology spoke to me about it. He explained that acetylcholine is released into the brain tissues during learning and is critical in acquiring new memories. It appears to make it easier for 'receptors' (technically called NMDA receptors) on the surface of brain cells to pass on messages between them, thereby improving intellect and memory. The Bristol team's vital discovery is that other areas on the surface of the same brain cells, called slow potassium channels (or SK channels), restrict the activity of these receptors, leading to poorer accumulation of new memories and knowledge.

Why is this so important? If the team can find drugs that enhance the NMDA activity and block SK activity, then these should boost both memory and intellect. In effect, they are looking for drugs that act like acetylcholine in the brain, but without its side effects. The way is open to stopping the deterioration of dementia, and perhaps even reversing it. Dr Mellor admitted to me that his team's findings will not revolutionize overnight the treatment of Alzheimer's disease, or of other causes of dementia or intellectual impairment, but they should lead to promising new ways of eventually doing just that. Progress in formulating new drugs has been accelerating dramatically in the last two decades, so we may expect specific treatments for intellectual impairment much sooner than we could have imagined a few years ago. If the treatment works, then the way is open to identifying people at high risk of dementia, or in its earliest stages, and using these new medicines to prevent or reverse it.

Alzheimer's genetics

If you have, or had, a close relative with Alzheimer's disease, it's natural to worry about the chances of developing it yourself. If it runs strongly in your family, you would be forgiven for thinking that nothing you can do will help you stave it off. You deduce that you are pre-programmed to have it and that, sadly, is that.

Recent reports, happily, don't support this. As in all diseases that seem to be passed from one generation to another, there is much more to this than inheritance. In the nineteenth century, doctors were convinced that tuberculosis was an inherited disease because there were families all the members of which had it. Of course, this was because it was infectious, and close contact between parents and children, and between siblings, spread the bacterium causing it.

Dementia isn't infectious, as far as we know, but there are other aspects of family living that may provoke cases in relatives, that are little to do with their genetics. They share the same environment, and this may lead to the wrong eating habits, or poor early education, or tobacco and alcohol habits, perhaps leading to violence, all of which may provoke dementia in later life. So the fact that one member of a family has dementia doesn't mean that others in the same family will develop it too. They may share the same genes, but their social habits and environment may change as they become adult, and that may make a difference.

Where you live does seem to matter. In some countries (such as parts of Finland and Italy), Alzheimer's disease has been reported as more common in women than in men. In others, such as the UK, Sweden, Japan and other areas of Finland, it attacks the sexes equally. Among the Cree in North America, Alzheimer's is reported to be extremely rare.

We don't know why these differences exist – if indeed they do, because they may arise from artefacts in data collection. Doctors may differ from country to country in the ways they record and diagnose Alzheimer's.

So are there families in which dementia occurs far more often than the norm? In every family in which a case is diagnosed it is natural for the relatives to ask about their chances of getting it too. This may be the reason you have started to read this book. I'll try to give an answer that will help you resolve your worries.

A history of dementia in a first-degree relative (parent or sibling) does mean that you have slightly more chance of developing it yourself than has a person with no such history. But that shouldn't worry you: as dementia is quite rare in people under 80 years old, you still have little chance of developing it until you are very old. And remember, these statistics were gathered from life tables in previous generations: your chances of avoiding dementia are better now, because we are aware of the factors in our lifestyles that promote it, and can therefore avoid them.

In the whole of Europe there are only a few recorded families (they number fewer than 20) in whom the dominant inheritance of a gene carrying a susceptibility to dementia leaves members with a one in two chance of eventually dying from the disease. You will know if you have the misfortune to be in one of them; none of them are in the UK.

One group of people, sadly, is an exception to this lack of obvious inheritance of Alzheimer's disease. Nearly all people with Down's syndrome develop amyloid plaques and neurofibrillary tangles by the time they are 40 years old, and with them they have the symptoms of dementia. The clue to their misfortune is found on chromosome 21.

Chromosomes are the strings of proteins on which we 'thread' our genes, of which we have many thousands. Genes produce the characteristics that make us unique: our eye and hair colour, our height, much of our appearance, our immune system, and so on. We have 23 pairs of 'somatic' chromosomes that determine almost all our bodily characteristics apart from our gender. That is decided by our sex-determining pair of chromosomes (labelled XX or XY).

Down's syndrome arises because of a mutation in a specific position on chromosome 21: it lies immediately beside another gene, mutation in which causes early onset Alzheimer's disease (which starts before the age of 50). The link between Down's syndrome and Alzheimer's dementia is that the mutation may involve the whole segment of the chromosome that involves both genes. People with one mutation are more likely than usual to possess the other one, too.

Geneticists have linked at least three other mutations with Alzheimer's disease, on chromosomes 1, 14 and 19. The one on chromosome 19 was a clue to identifying an underlying biochemical fault in Alzheimer's disease. The gene involved is linked to the production of a substance, a combined fat and protein, called apolipoprotein E, or ApoE. There are several types of ApoE, separated by subtle differences in their chemistry. Inheriting one of them, ApoE4, from both parents, giving a 'double ApoE4', has been linked to a seventeen-fold increase in a person's risk of Alzheimer's disease. This is frightening stuff, and has led in some countries to a demand for testing their healthy populations for it. It was suggested that the differences in rates of Alzheimer's between countries might be due to their different rates of possession of the ApoE4 gene. However, much more recent surveys of factors leading to dementia have suggested that possession of the double ApoE4 gene is not nearly as decisive as environmental and lifestyle factors, about which you will read more later.

Studies of chromosome 14 suggested that a gene on it that released substances called 'heat shock proteins' might contribute to dementia – the idea being that they might initiate inflammatory changes in the brain that would lead to plaques and tangles. Amyloid precursor protein, the researchers found, is produced by a gene on chromosome 21, and it, too, has been the subject of research. If it were possible to block the formation of amyloid by disabling that gene, it might lead to arrest of the process of plaque formation.

None of these studies, however, should lead people to rush into getting their genes tested. There are 100-year-old people with double ApoE4 who are completely normal for their age, so there must be other factors that set off the disease. There are also people with Alzheimer's who do not possess any of the 'rogue' genetics. So far, genetic studies are only useful in finding pointers to future possible treatments, and not to predict who will, and who won't, get Alzheimer's.

We have to look for other ways than genetic manipulation if we are to try to prevent its onset.

Tau protein and metformin

Enter Professor of Molecular Medicine Susan Schweiger, of Dundee University's Division of Medical Sciences. She cycles to work alongside the River Tay, and she obviously does her best thinking at that time, before the pressures of the daily routine kick in. Ruminating on a possible link between poorly controlled diabetes and dementia, it came to her on one of her cycle rides that the drug metformin, which has been used for many years to help people with Type 2 diabetes, might help prevent and even treat dementia.

We use metformin to control the blood glucose levels in diabetes, and until scientists like Professor Schweiger unravelled the mechanisms by which it does so, we didn't fully understand the links between the illness and dementia. The clue lay in the discovery that metformin increases the activity of an essential substance called protein phosphatase 2a, which is known to be almost absent in Alzheimer's disease. But the tale is more complicated (sorry!). Protein phosphatase 2a controls the production and activity of another protein called tau. Tau is present in all nerve cells, but it comes in several forms. The form of tau found in Alzheimer's disease appears to be abnormal, and is in some way linked to damage to the brain cells.

Professor Schweiger reasoned that if the abnormal tau could be reduced and normal tau levels substituted, the brain would be protected against the deterioration of Alzheimer's. Metformin might be the drug to do just that. It did so in cultures of nerve cells in the laboratory, and it was then tested in mice, strains of which also carry the same tau abnormality as Alzheimer's patients. It was a defining moment in her work. The mouse-brain normal tau levels improved.

Professor Schweiger has already started studies in humans and has applied for permission to conduct full large-scale trials in patients and people considered at high risk of dementia. She and her team propose that metformin will not only help to prevent diabetics from developing dementia, but that non-diabetics, too, will benefit from the drug. They do not expect improvement in nerve cells that have already died off through dementia, but they do suggest that it will prevent cells that are as yet undamaged by the disease from becoming affected.

Metformin will not be a cure for Alzheimer's disease, but it is the best bet yet for a medication that will stave off its effects. The big bonus is that it has been prescribed for diabetes for forty years, so that all its adverse effects are known and we can use it safely without the years of delay in toxicity testing that a completely new research drug would have to face.

There is one other advantage to metformin: as we have so many years of data from its millions of prescriptions, there may be scope for trawling through them to see if its protection against dementia is hidden among them. Among people who have taken it for years, are there fewer cases of Alzheimer's disease? Some keen PhD or MD student is bound to take that subject as a thesis. It could be a medical blockbuster. Professor Schweiger's work was published in the *Proceedings of the National Academy of Sciences* of the USA in November 2010. Her message won't be missed.

In the meantime there is nothing to stop doctors prescribing metformin for people in the earliest stages of Alzheimer's disease. Until we know more about it, however, it is probably not yet time to give it to everyone who is thought to be at risk but has not yet developed any sign of the illness.

Glivec and amyloid

Metformin is not the only current drug already prescribed for another disease that holds some promise for preventing Alzheimer's. Nobel Prize winner Professor Paul Greengard, Director of the Fisher Center for Alzheimer's Research at Rockefeller University in New York, reported in September 2010 that the antileukaemia treatment imatinib (Glivec) may prevent the build-up of amyloid.

However, we won't be able to use Glivec itself to prevent or cure dementia. One reason for that is that when given by mouth it doesn't get across the barrier between the bloodstream and the brain. Its formula will have to be manipulated to achieve that. Another objection is that Glivec has many serious side effects: they can be tolerated when the person's illness is immediately life-threatening, but not for people in good health who wish to prevent a disease that they may never develop.

So why does Professor Greengard see it as a hopeful development for dementia? The formation of amyloid between brain cells, already mentioned as a crucial part of Alzheimer's, depends on a protein called GSAP. The professor's team found that Glivec binds chemically to GSAP, blocking its action. Without active GSAP, there is no amyloid and therefore, hopefully, no Alzheimer's-type dementia.

So far, all the work has been done on mice. Mice bred not to make GSAP develop far fewer amyloid deposits in their brains than mice with normal GSAP levels. Professor Greengard sees this as good grounds for developing drugs that act like Glivec on amyloid production, that will cross into the brain after being swallowed and that would have minimal side effects. It may seem fanciful, but the theory is good and, with techniques in new drug development improving year by year, it is a strong contender for future dementia prevention.

Vitamin B and dementia prevention

What about the vitamin B story that I mentioned in the Introduction? Was there a reasonable basis for it? It came from a very respectable team of researchers from Oxford and from Norway. They subjected 168 volunteers over 70 years old to MRI scans of the brain over two years. All the volunteers were known to have memory problems but not severely enough to be diagnosed with dementia. MRI accurately measures the size of the brain, so that the repeated scans measured any shrinkage of the brain substance over the time of the study. Brain shrinkage correlates very well with other measures of severity of dementia – the faster the brain shrinks, the more severe the dementia.

During the study the subjects were given either tablets containing vitamins B_6 and B_{12} (two of the 12 forms of vitamin B) or a placebo vitamin look-alike containing no active ingredients. The researchers described the differences between the two groups at the end of the study as 'very striking' and 'dramatic'. The vitamins appeared to slow brain shrinkage by an average of 30 per cent, and in some cases (those with the most initial shrinkage) by more than 50 per cent.

Professor David Smith, of Oxford University's Department of Pharmacology, stated that the effect was much greater than the team had expected. He hoped that vitamins B_6 and B_{12} might delay the development of Alzheimer's disease in many people with mild memory problems. However, there was a caveat: we still do not know if there are drawbacks to taking them long term, and evidence from previous well-controlled and statistically evaluated trials of other vitamin supplements (of A and E) suggests that they may have serious disadvantages. Not only did they fail to improve health, but also they led to an even higher than expected death rate from all causes, particularly cancer.

So I would definitely not recommend that you start taking vitamin supplements. However, that is not a bar to eating foods high in vitamin B_6 and B_{12}. Among them are legumes such as beans and peas, meat and liver, wholegrain cereals and breads, and bananas. In effect, eat a wide variety of foods and you should at least cover the vitamin aspect of your protection regimen against dementia!

Vascular dementia

Alzheimer's is primarily a disease in which the brain cells die off. Why they do so isn't yet known precisely, although there are plenty of theories, but it is accepted that the primary failure is in the brain cells themselves. It is the cause of two-thirds of all cases of dementia in the developed world.

Most of the remaining third are caused by problems in the blood flow to the brain, leading to parts of the brain surface being deprived of oxygen. This is defined as 'vascular' dementia, and the commonest way in which it develops is in a series of 'mini-strokes'. The primary cause of vascular dementia is long-term damage to the arteries in the brain: its consequence is loss of the brain cells beyond that damage, because they have lost their blood, and there-fore oxygen, supply.

We know much more about the causes and background of vascular dementias than we do about Alzheimer's. That doesn't necessarily mean that it is easier to manage, but at least we can give guidance on its prevention to people whom we can identify to be at risk of it years before it arises. If you have uncontrolled high blood pressure, smoke, have the wrong type of blood lipid (fat) pattern, are considerably overweight and have known diabetes, you are at risk. If you know that one or more of these risk factors applies to you, then the rest of this book applies to you. Please carry on reading!

Whether or not you eventually get vascular dementia depends largely on how well you look after your circulation. If you can keep the inside surface of your blood vessels and your heart as smooth as possible, with no deterioration or damage, you are much less likely to have microscopic clots forming on them that can be the focus for developing larger clots, which then can break up and be scattered into the brain. This is the way in which multiple mini-strokes form, and it is from multiple mini-strokes that dementia develops.

The inside surface of blood vessels is a single layer of cells called the endothelium. A normal endothelium controls the passage of nutrients and oxygen from the blood across it into the tissues. It also controls the passage in the reverse direction of waste products of metabolism and carbon dioxide from the tissues into the bloodstream. So it is a pretty special organ, which if unrolled into a flat surface would cover a couple of football fields.

The problem is that, like the surface of a professional football field, any small defects in it can lead to harm that is out of proportion to their size. A hole in the turf can break an ankle or disable a knee. A small patch of porridge-like deterioration in an artery can lead to a heart attack or a stroke. An area of roughness in one of the coronary arteries can lead to a heart attack. A clot in one of the chambers of the heart, or a patch of degeneration in one of the carotid arteries leading to the brain, can give rise to multiple small clots that block what we call end-arteries in the brain, and to the main cause of vascular dementia.

At the time of the Korean War, US Army pathologists examined the endothelium of young men who had tragically been killed in the fighting. Most were between the ages of 18 and 22 years. Most already had signs of deterioration in their endothelium that were the start of the process that would have eventually led to heart attacks and strokes if they had lived into early old age. Many of them would have experienced vascular dementia.

If we are to prevent ourselves from developing this type of dementia, we therefore need to start years before it impinges on our lives – preferably in our childhood, but definitely in our early and middle adult years. I will return to this theme in more detail later in the book.

Telling the difference – Alzheimer's vs vascular

Faced with someone with dementia, a GP needs to decide its type. Is it Alzheimer's or vascular? The treatment depends on which it is: Alzheimer's needs drugs that will hopefully help the nervous system, and vascular dementia requires close attention to the difficulties in the patient's circulation, such as dealing with clots and keeping blood vessels open.

Recognition that the two illnesses have different onsets and patterns of progression led New Yorker Professor Hachinski to devise his scale for differentiating between the two. It allocates numbers to sections such as abrupt onset; progression in steps rather than gradually; physical complaints; emotional swings; past or current high blood pressure and stroke; and signs of nerve problems such as temporary blindness, weakness or numbness. A Hachinski score of 0 to 4 suggests Alzheimer's; one of 5 to 10 suggests vascular dementia or perhaps both.

Table 1 overleaf shows the scale. It is not perfect. Using it over the years I've found that many patients with dementia show elements of both types of disease, so making the definitive diagnosis is often academic. However, people with scores suggesting an element of vascular dementia need treatment for their circulation problems. It may mean simply adding an aspirin (to prevent blood clotting) and a blood pressure-lowering agent, but it matters. Neglecting to do so may mean a more rapid descent into end-stage dementia.

Table 1 The Hachinski scale

Symptom	Score
Sudden onset	2
Stepwise deterioration	2
Physical complaints	1
Emotional swings	1
Past high blood pressure	1
Past stroke	1
Neurological symptoms (pins and needles, dizziness)	2
Neurological signs (numbness, weakness, paralysis)	2

A score of 0 to 4 suggests Alzheimer's disease; from 5 to 10 indicates vascular dementia or both.

Two cases

Perhaps a better way to compare the two main types of dementia is with two fairly typical cases. Earlier I mentioned Jean, the 59-year-old teacher with Alzheimer's. Sadly she is now in her final stages within ten years of her diagnosis: many Alzheimer's sufferers last much longer. The natural history of the disease can be two decades long, most of which is spent in dependency on family and professional carers.

Roger

Take the case of Roger, the managing director of a company supplying specialist products to large-scale manufacturers. In his late fifties, he was on the top of his game; his company was successful, winning contracts all over the UK and Europe. I met him for the first time at a dinner party, when I was surprised to hear him tell the same funny story three times during the evening, once at the table, then later as we were sitting around recovering from our overeating, and last thing, when we were going for our cars.

The experience disturbed me. He hadn't had too much to drink and he appeared normal in every other way. I happened to be the regular locum for his doctor, so the next time I was on duty I told her about it. She was surprised, as she had no inkling that anything was wrong with him. He had attended a 'well man' clinic a few months before and had been given a clean bill of health. No high blood pressure, and none of the tests showed anything abnormal. She had not considered dementia or alcoholism (another strong cause of people repeating themselves). However, she knew his wife better, and would tactfully inquire after her husband's health when she saw her at a routine follow-up for a minor illness in the next two weeks.

My colleague called me after that appointment. His wife had noticed that Roger wasn't as 'sharp' as he used to be. Being managing director, he had been able to delegate the important decisions for his company to his managers, and at home she made all the domestic decisions. She had been hiding her fears about his mental capacity, but was now glad that they were out in the open.

His doctor called him in on a pretext, engineered by his wife, that he needed a medical for insurance. He was happy to oblige, and he underwent a series of mental tests that showed how far down the dementia line he had slipped. His short-term memory was very poor, and when asked about such common knowledge as the dates of the Second World War or the name of the monarch or the US president, he prevaricated. He was unable to repeat a series of seven numbers forwards or five numbers backwards. His Mini Mental State Examination score, a measure of the depth of dementia, was well in the range of Alzheimer's of several years' standing.

Roger retired early. He remained comfortable at home, affable, untouched apparently by his diagnosis. Over the next few years his wife looked after him, and once a week his golfing friends took him out for a day to give her a break. Ten years after that first ominous dinner party, I met him again. He was sitting in our golf clubhouse with his mates, calmly drinking a pint of beer. He looked up at me and smiled, but did not speak. I'm sure he didn't know who I was.

His three pals invited me to sit beside them. They told me that he hadn't spoken for a year, and that they had to do everything for him. They were glad to help him and his wife. He still made up the four for a round of golf every week. They had to put the right club in his hands, and count his score for him, but he could still win a few holes. His golf swing and his putting skills hadn't deserted him, even though he had lost everything else.

It was an amazing story, but no more amazing than that of the university lecturer, who, ten years after his early retirement with a diagnosis of Alzheimer's, could still complete the difficult cryptic crossword in *The Guardian* every day, long after he no longer knew his own children.

Alzheimer's is a strange illness, conserving some parts of the brain but not others, and it shows in such tragic cases.

Margaret

Margaret was a successful and highly talented secondary schoolteacher who accepted a headship when she was 50. It was a huge school, with nearly 2,000 pupils, and needed every ounce of dedication and application for her to keep on top of the job. This she did for eight years, but at the expense of 30 cigarettes a day and a share of a bottle of wine every night with her lawyer husband. With two good incomes and the children having fled the nest, they didn't stint themselves.

Margaret's doctor did warn her of burning the candle at both ends and in the middle but she didn't take his advice, especially on the cigarettes. 'They keep me sane,' she would tell him, as at each surgery visit he checked her rather poor control of her blood pressure.

He was surprised, however, when Margaret's husband came to him one day for advice about her. For the first time in her eight years at the school, the inspectors had given it a less than excellent report. It appeared that her teachers had been worried for some time about her temper and attitude to them. She had become forgetful and untidy, and her relations with the staff and even the children had worsened. These changes in her abilities and character had been sudden – she had turned from an impeccably effective manager to a termagant almost overnight.

Her doctor called her in for tests. She was reluctant to come but was persuaded by her husband. It turned out that her heartbeat was irregular, her blood pressure was high and, ominously, she admitted to short periods in the last few months in which she had lost her vision for a few seconds. From time to time she had been so dizzy that she had almost fallen. Although she was right-handed, she had taken to using her left hand for many of her kitchen chores because she felt her right hand was weak. She was still smoking 30 cigarettes a day, though she had cut her alcohol consumption to a glass of wine a day 'because I felt it was making me woozy'.

Her doctor arranged for her to see a vascular physician. Angiograms and brain scans showed that she had had multiple small strokes affecting the surface of her brain, probably arising from areas of degeneration in her carotid arteries. She was warned that she had to stop smoking and to cut her alcohol consumption to a single small glass per day, and that she should stop work.

She didn't (or couldn't) take the advice. She continued to smoke and drink, and the erratic behaviour continued. She was given prolonged leave of absence from the school on full pay. It didn't help. Month by month her deterioration became more obvious. She soon became unable to organize her domestic or monetary affairs. She could not go out without her husband, as she would get lost – in a town in which she had lived all her life. Her friends rallied round the couple as she rapidly lost all her social graces and, with them, her personality. Two years from the first diagnosis she died in a nursing home. Repeat brain scans over those years had shown many more small areas of destroyed brain-surface tissue, showing that the small strokes had continued, sometimes arriving in showers of clots.

Margaret had 'multi-infarct dementia': 'infarct' is our name for the death of tissue after its oxygen supply has been blocked. It was directly related to her smoking, about which much more later. Would she have survived longer if she had stopped smoking when asked to do so? It is difficult to say, as the damage had been done over many years and probably could not have been reversed. But there is no doubt that if she had never smoked she would never have suffered these two terrible years at the end of her too-short life.

Roger would have scored 0 on the Hachinski scale: Margaret's score was 9. They are not extreme cases; they are typical of Alzheimer's and vascular dementias that GPs like me have seen in practice over and over again. Alzheimer's disease usually takes longer than does vascular dementia to reach the end stage, but it is more difficult to slow and stop, and impossible to reverse. We can do much more for the early stages of vascular dementia, provided the person can co-operate and has an understanding of what can be done by working with his or her medical team. But they are not the only types of dementia: there are others that are more difficult to prevent or influence.

Other dementias

Around 10 per cent of dementias can't be classified simply as typical Alzheimer's or vascular. Medically, they are classified as:

- diffuse Lewy body disease
- fronto-temporal dementia (including Pick's disease)
- alcohol-induced dementia
- post head-injury dementia
- dementia linked to Parkinson's disease
- AIDS-related dementia
- Creutzfeldt-Jakob dementia
- Huntington's dementia.

Diffuse Lewy body disease is named after the microscopic changes seen in the brain, which differentiate it from all other types of dementia. We define it as the presence of dementia for at least six months, along with periods of confusion and hallucinations. People with Lewy bodies tend to 'see things' more than others with different dementias. They fall a lot and show odd neurological signs such as rigid muscles. They move much more slowly, and much less, than normal. They are often over-sensitive to drugs given for mental illnesses, and they deteriorate much faster than the average person with Alzheimer's.

People with fronto-temporal disease keep their memory until late in their illness. The main change is in their personality. They combine apathy with irritability, a strangely misplaced jocularity and cheerfulness, and lose their usual tactfulness and good manners, their concern for others, and their ability to make reasoned judgements and decisions in their business and private lives. Through all this, they have no insight into their often disastrous problems and mental state.

They find language difficult, so that they cannot recall important words in a conversation, making them 'talk round' a subject rather than addressing it directly. A well-known feature of fronto-temporal dementia is the constant repetition of anecdotes and jokes, which when it was first described in the mid-twentieth century gave it the name 'gramophone syndrome'. I'm not sure what it would be called now that 'gramophone' has disappeared from our language.

Unfortunately, another feature of fronto-temporal dementia is often an increased sex drive, which in view of the other personality changes is highly inappropriate.

Fronto-temporal dementia starts at a younger age than Alzheimer's and about one case in five is inherited. It includes a subset of patients with Pick's disease, in which the brain contains large 'ballooned' nerve cells first seen by a Professor Pick. However, most people with fronto-temporal dementia do not show Pick's changes in their brain.

The other types of dementia include that due to excessive alcohol (a cardinal sign in alcoholic dementia is Korsakoff's syndrome, in which the person constantly repeats statements, forgetting that he or she has made them only a few minutes before). This may be a fronto-temporal effect, as in the cases mentioned above. Huntington's disease is an inherited disease leading to early dementia. We are told that one person with Huntington's disease came to America on the *Mayflower* in 1620, and that it has affected more than 2,000 of his descendants. One may have been Woody Guthrie, the musician struck down with it in the 1940s. Dementia is the final stage in many cases of AIDS and in all cases of CJD, and Parkinson's disease carries with it a higher than normal risk of dementia. These are all special cases that need highly trained medical teams to cope with them, as do the more than a hundred other types of dementia that have been described in the medical journals. Most of them are single reports of particular syndromes linked to degeneration in a part of the brain. Their management remains the same as that of Alzheimer's disease.

The ageing gene – in worms and maybe in Henry

What about the idea that dementia isn't a disease after all, but an inevitable accompaniment of normal ageing? I'm not in favour of it as an idea, mainly because it is so depressing, leaving us with no possibility of avoiding it. People can reach advanced age with few signs of ageing. I regularly meet an old patient who has become a good friend over the many years we have known each other. We talk about old times, of course, but also about the new. We don't see completely eye to eye politically, but the arguments are softer now, and we do seem to be drawing closer on the essential things. Henry has kept his keen interest in what is going on in the UK and the rest of the world. He is still as sharp as he was as a young advocate arguing for justice in the courts and, later, dispensing it as a judge. He can still swing a golf club better than I can, though he needs a motorized cart to get him around the full 18 holes. He goes to a Qi Gong class once a week, is a keen member of our local discussion group, and is slim without being too thin. He drinks the odd glass of wine and has a whisky before going to bed, at around his usual time of eleven o'clock, though he admits to staying up for the finish of *Question Time* and maybe even for *This Week* (which takes him well past midnight).

Henry is 98 and looks twenty years younger.

What makes him so different from the rest of us? Does he have a secret that we need to know about?

I don't think so. Like many of his peers he fought through the war, part of it in Burma behind the Japanese lines with the Chindits. He entered law after the war, enjoyed good food and wines, and travelled a lot by motor bike, sustaining the odd head injury before crash helmets came into vogue. He smoked when young, stopping only in his fifties. He didn't, obviously, stop drinking. He has enjoyed a happy marriage: Elizabeth is 12 years his junior. He has had remarkably good health, the only blip being prostate enlargement in his seventies that our surgeon dealt with successfully.

So what is his advantage over the rest of us, for fewer than one in 1,000 of us will reach his age in such good mental and physical health?

Dr Robin May, of Birmingham University's Biotechnology and Biological Sciences Research Council, would probably say that Henry was born with an exceptionally fortunate variant of the DAF-16 gene.

Dr May is one of the UK's experts in ageing, but his evidence for the DAF-16 gene's role in determining how well or badly, or how fast or slowly, we age wasn't based on humans. The Birmingham team studies a laboratory worm that goes by the wonderful name of *Caenorhabditis elegans*, or *C. elegans* for short.

C. elegans is exceptionally useful in studying ageing, because DAF-16 is found in many other animals, including ourselves. Naturally worms age much faster than we do, so many generations of them can be assessed in a few years, and the results may reflect, in some way, what happens in human generations. What is fascinating about the Birmingham worms is that there are four separate species, with different types of DAF-16 activity. And their rate of ageing – how long the worms live – depends on which type they have inherited. DAF-16 also determines the way they react to stress (yes, you can put stress on a worm) and how immune they are to infections.

Dr May says,

> DAF-16 is part of a group of genes that drive the biological processes involved in ageing, immunity and responses to physical or environmental stresses. The fact that subtle differences in DAF-16 activity between species seem to have such an impact on ageing and health is very interesting, and may explain how differences in lifespan and related traits have arisen during evolution.

The Birmingham researchers are now studying how DAF-16 coordinates a complex network of genes to balance the different needs of an individual's immune system as he or she ages.

Professor Douglas Kell, a colleague of Dr May, says that the worm model is uncovering the biology of ageing, an essential preliminary to appreciating how older people's physiology changes as they become unwell or have difficulties with everyday tasks such as recalling memories or in moving around the home and elsewhere.

Although the worm is a very simple animal biologically, the research wasn't easy. The team followed four species of worm – they go under the wonderful names of *C. elegans*, *C. briggsae*, *C. remanei* and *C. brenneri*. *C. remanei* are the most fortunate in their DAF-16 activity, living much longer than the rest: their DAF-16 activity is 12 times greater than that of *C. elegans*. The researchers exposed the poor worms to heat, metallic poisons and bacterial and fungal infections. Those that expressed most DAF-16 lived the longest, and were more likely to live through the stresses and to recover from them fastest.

If you are cynical about the idea that what we find in worms is relevant to ourselves, don't be. Many of the genes we use for our immune systems and our ageing processes are similar to DAF-16. This is only the beginning of our understanding of ageing and why people like Henry are so good at it. If we do unravel the process, there's no reason why we couldn't help everyone to be like him.

2

Dementia in the UK – 2010

In September 2010 BBC prime-time news carried a report that 1 per cent of the national budgets – not simply the health budgets – of all developed countries is spent on the care of people with dementia. That was a surprise to me. As a doctor working in general practices with dozens of old and not-so-old people with dementia on their lists, my first reaction was that this wasn't excessive. However, when I took time to take in the financial burdens imposed by all the other demands on a nation's purse, I had to accept that it is a huge sum, and it is predicted to swell to triple its size in the next two decades. By that time the working population will be unable to support the financial and practical burden of dementia in all its forms. We have a desperate need to do as much as we can to prevent it now – yet we have little proven evidence on how to do so.

To be able to tackle the problem we must understand its extent. Surprisingly, the first comprehensive study of the survival of people with dementia cared for in general practice (in their own homes) in the UK was not published until 2010. Greta Rait and her colleagues of Birmingham University studied 22,529 people known to have dementia and 112,645 people without dementia between 1990 and 2007. Among all the statistics they collected about this massive study population, the one most crucial to us is that people diagnosed with dementia in their sixties live an average of 6.7 years; survival if diagnosed in their nineties is 1.9 years. In the first year after diagnosis their mortality is three times that of people of the same age without dementia.

These facts are bad enough, but hidden among them are even more unpalatable ones. At the time we GPs diagnose dementia, most people with it have been losing their abilities to reason, to understand and to remember things for years. That is why the death rate was so high in the Birmingham study: their diagnoses were mostly made only after the disease caused a crisis in care or late in its progression. So much dementia is hidden at home. If we are to prevent the worst aspects of dementia we must be able to diagnose it sooner and develop methods to slow it down or even, hopefully, to reverse it, long before it lands people in studies such as that of Dr Rait and her team.

Why is it so difficult to make the diagnosis earlier? Back to Elizabeth England again. She pinpoints the different ways that dementia shows itself, people's beliefs that there are no treatments for it even if they recognize that something is wrong, and lack of training and skills in recognizing the subtle signs of dementia even among health professionals such as GPs like me. We are not as efficient as we should be in differentiating between the changes in memory and understanding that happen with normal ageing and those of dementia.

In 2009 the UK Department of Health published the National Dementia Strategy, which has three aims – to raise awareness of dementia, to make its assessment easier and more widely available, and to improve dementia services. It hasn't been universally accepted. One objection is that it encourages doctors to refer patients to consultant services, when most dementia care takes place in the person's home and is run by GPs and their dedicated teams. Another objection is that for the strategy to work the treatments it employs should make a difference to the patients and carers: so far we don't have such treatments. That leads to disappointment and frustration, and the GPs, not the specialists, have to deal with them.

We in general practice are therefore faced with the need to spend more time with the families that are looking after relatives with dementia, to learn more about how to deal comprehensively with the problems that arise with dementia, to set up an efficient team of carers for each family, and to address when and if to initiate the care for the final stages of the illness. We can only do that if we have a good relationship with you, the carers and family. It isn't surprising, after all, that 1 per cent of each country's national budget is spent on one illness. Any improvement in its prevention would be an enormous saving in time, effort, stress and, most of all, suffering, not just for the patients themselves but for family and friends.

Can we prevent dementia?

So we need to try to prevent dementia. Popular health magazines have regular articles on how to do so. They all promote roughly the same messages – keeping fit physically and active mentally, eating healthily, avoiding bad habits, being sociable and outward-going, all the usual lifestyle messages. But do they actually work? Where is the statistically proven scientific and clinical evidence that any of these obvious and well-broadcast ideas actually make any difference to our chances of avoiding dementia? I hate to admit it, but it doesn't yet exist.

Here are Dr Karen Ritchie and her colleagues of the University of Montpellier and of St Mary's Hospital, London, on the subject. They managed to recruit 1,433 people chosen randomly from electoral rolls, all of them living at home, to a seven-year study. At the start they used a standard interview to assess their intellect and memory, their social status, nutrition and medical history, including exposure to anaesthetics, virus infections, asthma, diabetes, high blood pressure, stroke, heart disease, drug use, hormone replacement therapy (HRT) and depressive symptoms. Blood samples were taken to check on apolipoprotein Ee4 (about which more later), and fasting sugar and cholesterol levels.

After two, four and seven years Dr Ritchie's group reassessed the survivors for signs of dementia and related the results to each of the above factors. They picked out the ones that were most associated with dementia or its absence – and the results were surprising. The two that appeared to offer the greatest protection against dementia were a higher ability to read and high fruit and vegetable consumption. The factors most likely to increase the chance of developing dementia were depression and diabetes. The team concluded that the best chances of avoiding dementia lie in improving reading skills, eating fresh fruit and vegetables, curing depression and strictly controlling diabetes. All these lifestyle aspects were more important than possessing apolipoprotein Ee4, the genetic indicator commonly linked with higher than normal risk of developing Alzheimer's disease.

Dr Ritchie interpreted her group's findings warily. She did not rule out that the factors in her study that didn't seem to make a difference (such as high blood pressure, high cholesterol, previous anaesthetics, asthma, heart disease, HRT and drug use) might matter, but she concluded that increased reading ability, eating more fruit and vegetables, and controlling depression and diabetes would have the biggest impact on preventing dementia. She asked for researchers to pursue them in future studies.

Not everyone agreed with Dr Ritchie. Professor James C. Coyne, of the University of Pennsylvania, felt that concentrating on reducing depressive symptoms would be a poor way to prevent dementia. He argued that people become depressed for many reasons, many of them not medical. Depression can arise from social, economic and psychological causes, as well as from poor physical health not connected with dementia. If by controlling depression Dr Ritchie meant giving antidepressants, this, Professor Coyne argued, would be inappropriate. He warned that a similar argument had been put forward ten years previously, when depression was found to be linked with heart attacks, yet a huge trial in which depression was treated in post heart-attack patients did not show a reduction in their subsequent attack rate. He described a strategy of giving antidepressants to people in middle age with symptoms of depression just to prevent dementia as 'folly'.

This is strong stuff. Dr Chengxuan Qiu of the Karolinska Institute, Stockholm, went further. He wrote that Dr Ritchie and colleagues may be over-optimistic about programmes to prevent dementia, given the huge gap between theoretical programmes derived from observation and the findings from clinical trials. He added that while observational studies like Dr Ritchie's have often associated dementia with high blood pressure, high blood fat levels and diabetes, and have concluded that physical activity, good high blood pressure control and HRT potentially protect against its development, when trials testing these associations have been completed they have been inconclusive. He concluded that, so far, we do not have an effective intervention programme (for dementia prevention) for the general population.

So where does that leave us? Should we bother to try to prevent ourselves from developing dementia? Dr Qiu does have an answer.

His systematic review of all the studies shows that if we target people in middle age who have 'vascular' factors (such as high blood pressure) we should be able to reduce their risk of dementia. However, the target is not simply to reduce their blood pressure; Dr Qiu contends that we all need to target 'modifiable factors' (read Dr Ritchie's list again!) from midlife onwards to be effective in reducing our risk of dementia.

Which takes us round in a circle. So many lifestyle factors play a part in producing dementia in our last few years that we need to address them all. That is the only way we can best reduce our own personal risk of developing the disease. I am trying to do this myself – I'm not so young. The rest of the book is about how you can do so, too.

If you do, what are the chances that you might be successful in warding off dementia? Let's be optimistic and accept Dr Ritchie's calculations as being the most accurate we have so far.

Take the average 70-year-old with, so far, no dementia. I'm using the word 'we' here because I can't exclude myself:

- If we improve our literacy (Dr Ritchie used for this analysis the Neale adult reading test, which also includes an assessment of general knowledge), then we will cut our dementia incidence by 18 per cent.
- If we eliminate depression we improve our chances by 10 per cent.
- If we increase our fruit and vegetable consumption the gain is 6.5 per cent.
- And if we control diabetes we reduce dementia rates by 4.9 per cent.

The numbers are carefully calculated from her research findings; they are not plucked out of some geriatric hat. They may not seem big changes to someone outside medicine, but if they are correct they are a huge contribution to better health in older people. At least they are a start, though still an arguable one. If everyone succeeded in doing all four, the team estimated that the total burden of dementia in the community would fall by 21 per cent. Now we are talking in hundreds of thousands of cases over the years.

Naturally these figures have been put to the closest scrutiny. The *British Medical Journal* asked Tobias Kurth, Director of Research at the Hôpital de la Pitié-Salpêtrière in Paris, and Giancarlo Logroscino of the University of Bari, Italy, to review Dr Ritchie's work. They agreed that Dr Ritchie's study 'provides interesting information about the potential contribution of modifiable risk factors to the development of dementia'. However, they expressed doubts about how prevention programmes should be developed to eliminate these factors, who should be chosen for them, and for how long they should continue. They pointed out that a risk factor that may be harmful (promoting dementia) at a younger age, such as high blood pressure and high blood cholesterol levels, may in fact be protective in the old. 'In later life', they wrote, 'dementia is associated with lower blood pressure and lower cholesterol levels.'

They also stressed that although Dr Ritchie and her colleagues' study suggested that public health programmes to promote enhanced intelligence and increased fruit and vegetable consumption, and to treat depression and diabetes seriously should be a priority, there was lack of proof that they would do so. Instead, they concluded that because resources are limited, research should focus on whether only people at higher risk should be targeted for dementia-prevention resources. 'It is too early', they wrote (in August 2010), 'to call for general prevention programmes against dementia.'

So what can we conclude? If we were to follow Kurth and Logroscino's advice, we would do nothing. I prefer Dr Ritchie's way. As individuals, at any age, whether or not we are at extra risk of dementia, let's at least try her approach. If it hasn't been proven beyond doubt to prevent dementia, we can at least feel that we have done our best. Kurth and Logroscino offer us no alternative. So let's be optimistic and go for it.

3

Can we improve our brainpower – and will it help prevent dementia?

The transient fame of 'brain training'

It's common sense, isn't it, to conclude that if we improve our brainpower – our intellect, our ability to understand relatively complex things, and our memory – that the process should help us prevent our deterioration into dementia as we grow older. This was a theme much publicized in the later half of the first decade of our new century. It took off with many people buying into 'brain training' computer programmes, and praising them for improving memory and even intellectual performance.

The vogue for brain training was encouraged by Dr Joe Verghese and his colleagues at the Albert Einstein College of Medicine and Syracuse University, New York. They studied 469 subjects over the age of 75, all still living in their own homes. They recorded how much time they spent in leisure activities, their physical exercise levels and their thinking abilities, combining them all in a scoring system of 'activity-days per week'.

Over the next five years 124 of their 469 subjects developed dementia, 61 of whom had Alzheimer's, 30 vascular dementia and 25 mixed Alzheimer's and vascular dementia. Eight had less common causes of dementia. In a comparison of the activities of the dementia and non-dementia groups, it became clear that playing musical instruments, dancing, reading and playing board games all reduced the dementia risk.

The authors concluded that taking part in leisure activities is linked to a reduced risk of dementia, and suggested further studies be done to see how protective such activities that involve thinking are against its development. Dr Joseph Coyle, of Harvard Medical

School, wrote about the study in a 2003 editorial in the *New England Journal of Medicine*. He advised his doctor readers not to wait for further studies before putting its lessons into practice. 'Seniors', he wrote, 'should be encouraged to read, play board games, and go ballroom dancing, because, at the very least, they enhance their quality of life, and they might just do more than that.'

In my introduction to this chapter I mentioned common sense, and Dr Coyle's statement seems eminently one of common sense. Did the study not simply tell us what we already know, instinctively? Unfortunately, common sense and instinct are not necessarily correct. The huge flaw in the argument is that the subjects who eventually developed obvious dementia, and who had not been socially and physically active on entry to the study, might have had early dementia from the start – and that had made them less gregarious and less keen to learn new physical and mental skills. No amount of persuading them to play board games and dance would have made any difference to their descent into dementia.

Come 2010 and Dr Adrian Owen, who is pretty well qualified in the subject of brain function. He and his colleagues in the UK's Medical Research Council Cognition and Brain Sciences Group at Cambridge University didn't accept common sense as the final arbiter on whether or not brain training works. They asked more than 11,000 volunteers (30 times the number of subjects in the New York study) either to sign up to online brain training or simply to use the World Wide Web to answer a list of relatively difficult questions that Dr Owen and his team had set.

The results showed that the two groups did improve, equally, in their ability to perform the tasks they faced, but only in that one aspect. At the end of the study, whether they had been 'brain trained' or had simply surfed the web, neither group showed any improvement in intellectual performance or understanding – defined as their cognitive abilities. So, sadly, we have no evidence that brain training does us any lasting or even temporary good.

Be a musician

That doesn't mean, however, that nothing can help. The New York study had picked out one aspect of brain protection that has been confirmed in further work: playing a musical instrument. For as long as I can remember I have heard from different people whose judgement I trusted, including schoolteachers and tutors at medical school, that if we listen to classical music regularly it will help develop our brains and intellect in more ways than simply musical appreciation. As I'm not very musical, I found that advice hard to follow for myself, but the few professional musicians I know have all impressed me as being sharp and interesting people. Nevertheless, as someone who professes to follow the scientific method for my judgements, I put that old advice aside as anecdotal, rather than proven fact.

Now there is more than anecdotal evidence about music and the brain. A review of articles from such erudite journals as the *Journal of Neuroscience*, *Neuropsychologia*, *Nature Reviews Neuroscience* and *Psychological Science* comes down heavily in favour of using musical training to improve intellect. This is not anecdotal, and the evidence is impressive.

However, none of them suggests that simply listening to music does much for the brain – we have to be actively involved in music-making. Learning to play an instrument, as well as enriching our musical abilities, also improves memory, attention span, language skills and intellect, and makes us better, more rounded people. We become more empathetic to our fellow man and woman. These findings are based not on tests alone, but on changes in repeated brain scans. The younger we start our musical training, the better developed are the areas of our brain that deal with hearing and muscle movement and co-ordination. That is to be expected, but what wasn't expected in the studies was that the extra development of the brain occurs in areas not obviously involved directly with music.

For example, professional musicians have more grey matter, not just in the areas that we know relate to music-making, such as the control of fine movement and hearing, but also in the way we see things around us and how we fit in with them – a process the neurologists call visuo-spacial processing. This is something that I haven't yet shared with my close friend and neighbour, Rory Boyle, who is a well-known composer and lecturer at the Royal Scottish Academy of Music and Drama. I don't want him to feel too superior to me – I have never managed to master anything more than a toy drum, and that not too well.

Grey matter, the mass of nerve cell bodies and nerve fibres, deals with the spread and co-ordination of messages throughout the brain, and is directly related to intellect. Being professionally absorbed in playing and composing music from an early age appears to develop the grey matter, and the efficiency of the messages that flash through it, especially well.

I'll give you a clue about Rory – his opera *Kaspar Hauser* won him the prestigious Stage Works category of the British Composer Awards 2010. He also completed in 2010 his work for eight grand pianos and 16 pianists. In my book, you can't get more complex problems to solve than to make every note in a 32-hand piano piece gel – and he has done it brilliantly. Buy his CDs and wonder at why geniuses like him are not much better known to the general public.

In particular, musicians who began their instrumental training as children before they were seven years old, when the brain is still developing, have a thicker corpus callosum than we ordinary mortals. That is the area of the brain that communicates between its two halves. It is the same part of the brain that was found to be especially well developed in London cabbies after their study for 'the Knowledge', and is highly correlated with increased intellect, so even if you are older than seven (and as you are reading this book, you presumably are), you can still improve.

Changes in the brain are all very well, but are musicians, in general, any brighter than the rest of us? Sadly for the relationship between me and my composer friend, the answer seems to be yes. Trained musicians do have much better memories than the rest of us for lists of words spoken to them. They are far more able than the rest of us to remember sounds, and can concentrate for longer and more effectively on tasks that involve listening and hearing. Schoolchildren who play instruments can read better and have wider vocabularies than their non-musical peers. It has been proposed that training children early to play an instrument increases their intelligence quotient (IQ).

This isn't fanciful. Dr Patrick Ragert and his colleagues at the Ruhr University in Germany found, unsurprisingly, that professional pianists are far better than the rest of us in being able to discriminate two adjacent points (a standard test of spatial perception), and they can improve on this ability the more they practise on their instruments. This, according to Dr Ragert's team, means that the brain can adapt to improve its function, even in adults, and that learning an instrument improves other skills apart from the sole one of musical ability. If adults can do this, it should be even more obvious in children.

For example, on the whole musicians are better at learning foreign languages than non-musicians. That's especially true of tonal languages such as Mandarin and Cantonese, in which subtle changes in the sound of vowels make big changes in a word's meaning. Psychologists go even further: they suggest that because musical training involves recognizing the finer emotions expressed in sounds such as song or instrumental pieces, musicians, be they children or adult, are somehow more sympathetic to their fellows and mix more easily with them.

So is there an age beyond which playing music no longer improves our brainpower? Am I too late, at my advanced age, to make a difference to my own brain? Apparently not. We know that the earlier a child starts, the greater the enhancement in brain activity, but according to Dana Strait of Northwestern University, Illinois, there is good evidence that music training works at any age, including later life. That fits with the London taxi driver evidence; after all, they don't start to learn 'the Knowledge' until they are adults.

Does this mean that we should all try to learn a musical instrument to improve our chances of avoiding dementia? In my case I might not become demented, but I would probably be murdered by my long-suffering (and very musical) wife.

Bathe in the light

So what else can we do to improve our brain capacity? Here is a second surprise for those who found the musician effect a tad far-fetched: sit in bright light. Having light impinge on our eyes isn't simply about seeing. It lights up, if you will forgive the phrase, other parts of the brain apart from the one at the back that deals with vision – the visual cortex.

When people of normal intellect and eyesight were given tasks to perform and tests to complete, their results were far better if they were in very bright light when doing so. They were better able to find things (which may be stating the obvious), of course, but they also performed better at maths problems, were more efficient at using logic and reasoning to solve problems, and even their reaction times were faster than if in normal lighting. It seems that being in bright light makes us more alert – in effect 'geeing up' our brain.

Some of the studies about light verge on the incredible. When people were exposed to different colours of light during brain scans, it took only seconds for a response from the area of the brain known to make us alert. Blue light was the most powerful stimulant of this reaction.

Why should this happen? We have a pigment in our retina (the screen at the back of the eyes that reacts to light to allow us to see) called melanopsin. It has nothing to do with our visual mechanisms, but the researchers suggest that it specifically absorbs pale blue light, and that has something to do with the boost to our reasoning abilities. So should we lie in bright light as often as we can? We can only wait for long-term studies to confirm these early research findings. It occurs to me that if the connection is a true one, people living in the tropics should have a lower rate of dementia than the rest of us. However, there are so many causes of dementia that may be exclusive to the social deprivation of the Global South that no hard and fast conclusion can be drawn. It is easier to switch on plenty of light in our homes here than to emigrate to sunnier climes.

4

We are what we eat – or are we?

Eating for the brain

So we have started the musical instrument and are sitting in bright light (without shades). What else can we do to improve our brain-power? Will going on a special diet do the trick? Are there foods that will help develop the brain and prevent it going into free fall in our sixties, apart from the vitamin B-rich foods mentioned in Chapter 1?

Oily fish and omega-3

You are now entering a minefield. Who in the early twenty-first century has failed to be assailed by the promoters of omega-3 fatty acids? How many of us today don't accept that oily fish and certain green vegetables will benefit our brains, our hearts, our circulation and almost every other aspect of our health? They are added to so many foods that we feel uneasy about passing a day without swallowing our measured amounts of omega-3. In my *Guardian* mailbag for the 'Doctor, Doctor' column, hardly a week goes by without someone worrying about whether he or she is getting enough omega-3.

Is omega-3 really the panacea that it seems to be? Well, I'm not sure. It has been promoted solidly since the early 1980s, so more than three decades later we should have all the evidence we need to make a judgement on it. Sadly, we don't.

The name 'omega-3' covers a small group of fatty acids, the main ones being eicosapentaenoic acid (EPA) and docosahexaenoic acid (DHA). EPA has anti-inflammatory properties and DHA is essential for the structure of many types of cells in the brain, including the retinas in our eyes. Our main source of both is seafood, particularly oily fish. Basically, the idea that omega-3 is good for us comes from the discovery by Sir John Vane that we form prostacyclin, a substance known to prevent blood clots, from eating foods rich in it. The theory was that as blood clots are the main cause of heart attacks and strokes, foods containing plenty of omega-3 should protect against them.

By 1985 Dr Daan Kromhout had shown (in the *New England Journal of Medicine*, volume 312, page 1205) that eating even just a little more fish than the rest of the population will lower our risk of heart attacks and strokes. That opened the floodgates: study after study confirmed that eating foods rich in omega-3 reduces our chance of a second heart attack after we have had our first one.

We all started to eat oily fish or to take supplements of omega-3, until the inevitable letdown appeared in 2006. A review of all the published studies failed to confirm the benefits. The University of East Anglia team led by Dr Lee Hooper, whose conclusions spoiled the omega-3 party, were unrepentant. One of the studies, for example, had shown that men with angina who took fish oil supplements had a higher death rate than men who were taking only a placebo or were actually eating the fish, rather than the supplements.

The ball bounced back in 2008, with a huge combined report by the WHO and the UN Food and Agriculture Organization (FAO), which stated that taking fish oils or fish oil supplements for two years after a heart attack reduced the risk of another attack by about 18 per cent. Dr Hooper is relatively unimpressed. In an interview with *New Scientist* writer Sanjida O'Connell in May 2010 (issue 2760) Dr Hooper stated that 'we don't have good enough evidence' to prove the case for omega-3.

What has this to do with omega-3 and the brain? Let me introduce Durham County Council to you in the shape of Dr Madeleine Portwood, with Dr Alex Richardson from Oxford University. Their first study compared the use of a placebo and omega-3 fish oil supplements in almost 300 children. They concluded that the supplements improved the children's abilities to read, write and concentrate, but only in 40 per cent of the group. The second study's conclusion was that children who took omega-3 supplements before they sat their GCSE examinations achieved higher grades than those who didn't. It led to thousands of children taking the supplements, despite the fact that the study had a huge flaw – it had no placebo control group.

Since then, no one has produced a paper that confirms these remarkable benefits to the brain. And in April 2010 a two-year-long double-blind placebo-controlled study involving 867 people aged from 70 to 80 found no difference between takers of omega-3 and of placebo in tests of reasoning and understanding, defined as their cognitive ability.

Sadly – because it would be a very easy way to protect our brains against dementia if we could just take a supplement – the omega-3 bubble for improving our brainpower seems to have burst. We need to look elsewhere for a dietary protective factor.

Aside from omega-3, what about fish in general?

Should we forget all the hype about oily fish and omega-3, and look at fish in general? After all, one of the most persistent old wives' tales, promulgated for generations before omega-3 hit the headlines, was that if we ate fish we would improve our brainpower. Weren't we all told that as children – when the last thing we wanted to eat was fish?

Dr Joseph Hibbein, a psychiatrist working at the US National Institutes of Health in Bethesda, Maryland, promotes a more modern line that fish is good for our brains, particularly in dealing with depression and in reducing aggression. The overall rate of depression in a country, he says, is closely linked to the population's average consumption of fish. It doesn't need to be oily – his statistics don't differentiate between white fish and the oily kind. For example, he says, Japanese adults eat 12 times as much fish in a year (65 kilograms) as do Germans (under 5 kilograms). Depression affects one in 100 Japanese and one in five Germans.

The problem, of course, is that there may be other reasons why so many Germans and so few Japanese are diagnosed with depression, apart from their fishy (or non-fishy) habits. It isn't reasonable to accept that there is a cause and effect just because there is a statistical connection. However, if eating fish regularly does lift or prevent depression, it may be one key (among many others) to preventing eventual dementia. Depression through the early and middle adult years does seem to be linked to eventual dementia, although not in a straightforward and easily explicable way.

Flavonoids

Do flavonoids fit the bill? These are substances found in a fairly wide range of fruits, such as blackcurrants, blueberries and blackberries (brambles for my Scots readers), and in green tea, red wine and cocoa. Flavonoids hit the headlines in the early 1980s, when foods rich in them were claimed to prevent early deaths from heart attacks and strokes. The popular press have hailed them as today's panacea.

Do they work? Tests in laboratory rats showed that rats given extra flavonoids had better memories (they remembered better how to get out of a maze, for example) than rats given ordinary rat food. Their brains showed less degeneration than those of their peers. However, rats aren't humans.

Dr Jeremy Spencer of Reading University has advanced beyond experiments in rodents into early studies in human volunteers. He reported that eating blueberries in amounts that were equivalent to those given to the rats improved his subjects' attention span, and that blood tests showed that the flavonoids promoted the activity of genes involved in memory.

To summarize Dr Spencer's work, flavonoids should have several benefits for the protection of the brain against dementia. They increase brain levels of 'brain-derived neurotrophic factor', which enhances memory and learning, and they improve blood flow through the brain by relaxing the muscles in blood-vessel walls and decreasing blood pressure. They may even stimulate the growth of new nerves and connections within the brain by stimulating brain stem cells. All these effects should help the brain resist the degeneration that produces dementia.

Dr Spencer is obviously an enthusiast. Other scientists are a little more reticent about flavonoid benefits, feeling that we would need to eat vast amounts of flavonoid-containing foods to offer significant protection against dementia. However, most of them do seem to eat plenty of these foods themselves, in the hope that at the least they will do no harm, and may well do good. So red wine, black soft fruits, green tea and cocoa are the flavour of the times for the scientists in the know.

Magnesium

Older family doctors like myself were intrigued by the news in 2010 that magnesium might improve our brainpower. It came from the prestigious Massachusetts Institute of Technology in a report by Dr Guosong Liu and his team, who had fed a magnesium-containing compound to rats. They correlated the high levels of magnesium that it induced in the brain with improved memory, for both the space around them and repeated tasks that they had to perform. The magnesium-fed rats' brains also showed a significant increase (over brains in non-treated rats) in new nerve cell formation in the hippocampus – about which more later. Surprisingly, the improvement was just as noticeable in older as in younger rats, suggesting that even the older brain could benefit from the extra magnesium in the diet. It is enough to state here that a bigger, better hippocampus is related to higher intellect in humans. Dr Liu and his team extrapolate from the rodent experiments that magnesium supplements might improve our brains, especially in intellect.

Why should older family doctors be intrigued with this news? For decades we dosed many of our patients with magnesium-containing antacids, in amounts that would surely have increased their brain levels of the metal. I didn't notice any improvement in their intellectual capacity, and I'm fairly sure that is the experience of the rest of my British GP colleagues. However, we will wait for further studies to be done, first in volunteers and then, perhaps, in patients already showing some deterioration. I'm happy to take flavonoids, but I'm not sure about magnesium supplements, yet.

Starving ourselves

Could it be that we have been targeting the wrong area of our eating habits? Instead of adding foods to our daily menus, should we be subtracting them? Should we eat far less than we would really like to, leaving ourselves half-starved every day? We have known for years that laboratory rats live much longer than their peers if they are severely restricted in what they eat. It was taught to my generation of medical students, now a long time ago, that underweight animals are healthier animals that outlive their fatter cousins – and our teachers naturally assumed that this could be a lesson in healthy living for us.

The message of constantly semi-starving ourselves in order to extend our old age by a few years didn't appeal to our generation of impoverished students, and it hasn't been taken on in the general population, either. A few times a year I talk to primary schoolchildren about healthy living, and show them my old school photograph from the 1950s. It's one of those in which the pupils were arranged in a huge semi-circle and the camera rotated, so that they appear in a straight line. I ask the schoolchildren of today what makes the children then so different from now, and they talk about the short trousers, the ties and blazers, the haircuts, but never about the most obvious change. Among the 450 boys aged from 11 to 18, there is not a single one who is obese, or even slightly overweight. Yet in every class today, in every school, three or four of the children are already too heavy.

Even more startling are football crowds. I show the children football crowds from the 1960s: there isn't a single obese man among them. The thin schoolchildren have patently become thin adults. Now look at the crowds of today: it is hard to spot a thin spectator among many thousands. It is a colossal change in our population, and bodes ill for the future. The USA is ahead of us in the obesity stakes. It is estimated that in the next twenty years 40 per cent of US citizens will be clinically obese. That is, not just overweight, but overweight by so much (20 per cent or more) that their life expectancy is reduced by around ten years.

Allowing ourselves to eat so much that we become obese, therefore, allows us to avoid dementia by dying before we reach the age at which it begins. However, that isn't the aim of this book! What is the evidence that eating too little, so that we stay thinner than the norm, does the opposite? Will it really let us survive into a healthy and active old age, just like the laboratory rats?

As usual there are two opinions on this. July 2010 was the occasion of the annual conference of the British Society for Research on Ageing. It was held in Newcastle upon Tyne, a highly appropriate venue as Newcastle University is the home of the Centre for Integrated Systems Biology of Ageing and Nutrition, or CISBAN.

CISBAN researchers confirmed that laboratory animals whose food intake is restricted do live longer than others fed a standard diet judged enough to keep them a healthy, average weight. More importantly, they think they have discovered why they do so.

To understand their work, we first have to know about the ageing process. All through our lives the cells that make up our organs and tissues are constantly dying off and being replaced by younger versions. For example, some cells, such as our white blood cells and gut lining cells, may last only a few days. Others, such as red blood cells, last for months before being replaced, and bone cells survive for years before dying off. Until recently we thought that the nerve cells in our brains were never replaced when they died off, so that after the end of our brain growth in late childhood we would gradually have fewer and fewer brain cells until we died of old age.

When we learned what the ageing process is really about, these ideas had to be changed radically. Ageing starts at the cellular level. All our cells, of whatever type and in every organ, begin their lives by a process called mitosis, in which our 23 pairs of chromosomes line up and divide to form the nuclei of the new cells. At the end of each chromosome is a 'telomere', a structure that is thought to protect against errors occurring during mitosis that might lead to diseases. Unfortunately, as we age, each time a cell replicates itself the telomeres shorten a little, so that eventually there is hardly any telomere left. At that stage the cell can no longer replicate, and it dies. This is cell senescence.

We are born with longer or shorter telomeres: those of us with longer telomeres have the potential to live longer than those who have shorter telomeres. Anything we can do to keep our telomeres from 'eroding' will help us to live longer, and probably more healthily. We can get a good idea of how fast animals are ageing by examining the cells in the lining of the gut and the liver: masses of senescent cells, with shorter telomeres, means faster ageing and early death. The CISBAN team compared the numbers of senescent cells in the guts and livers of mice fed normally and those on a restricted food intake. There were far fewer senescent cells in the half-starved mice.

What fascinates doctors like me about this experiment is that the mice didn't have to be on a restricted diet from birth, or even from adolescence (yes, mice go through adolescence). Even if adult mice were fed less food for a relatively short time, the numbers of senescent cells were significantly reduced.

Dr Chunfang Wang, the head of the CISBAN team, proposed from their results that eating a very low-calorie diet helps to prolong lifespan. It reduces cell senescence and protects the telomeres from damage, and this in turn prevents the accumulation of damage in tissues that leads to diseases of ageing. One of these is dementia.

However, as always, we must be cautious in relating these mouse experiments to possible human benefit. Professor Thomas von Zglinicki, who oversaw the team's work, admitted that they did not yet know if food restriction delays ageing in humans, but at least the work shows that, if it does relate to humans, we can get some benefit if we start to eat less in later life. It may be an initial step towards knowing how to delay ageing in older people.

This tends to confirm the prejudice that many people have about obesity: that fatter people don't live as long as thin people. If you feel like that, then you have to face up to the fact that, so far, we haven't proved it. In fact, 2010 was the year that we had to face up to new facts about the hallowed measure of fatness and thinness – the body mass index, or BMI.

The BMI was established more than forty years ago as the standard by which we could judge whether adults were of normal weight for height, too light (too thin) or too heavy (overweight, obese or morbidly obese). Simply put, it is our weight in kilograms divided by the square of our height in metres. It was judged to be similar in men and women. So a man of 5 foot 10 inches (1.78 metres) weighing around 12 stone (76 kilograms) would have a BMI of about 23. This would be a normal weight for his height.

For years doctors have looked upon a BMI between 20 and 25 to be ideal – not too fat or too thin. Under 18, they understood, was so thin that there were health consequences. Between 25 and 30 we were overweight, between 30 and 40 we were obese, and above 40, morbidly obese – so fat that the condition severely limited life expectancy.

Now, with tables relating millions of BMI figures with life expectancy, we are revising these figures. It seems that the ideal BMI lies between 22.5 and 25, and that there is no difference in outlook between those with BMIs of 20 to 22.5 and those with BMIs of 25 to 27.5. They are only marginally worse off than the 'ideals'.

This is great news for the very many people who are just a little overweight (about a stone too heavy), but it is bad news for the CISBAN team. For whatever lifestyle people with BMIs of 22.5 to 27.5 have followed, it certainly doesn't include a restricted diet! And people who have starved themselves throughout their lives – with BMIs of 18 and under – die younger than their heavier counterparts. So it seems to be back to the drawing board on restricted diets. It does seem cruel, anyway, to impose a calorie-restricted diet on older people just to keep them alive a little longer. It would be sad to spend one's last years in the throes of hunger imposed by our doctor or carer just in the interests of living longer. If there were an extra advantage, such as if it kept our mental state in better fettle, there might be a reason for it – but that is by no means proven.

5

What do you think of it so far?
The NHS way to prevent dementia

So you have read this far and still don't really know the best ways for you to stave off dementia. You don't play a musical instrument, and the rest of the evidence so far in the hunt for strategies for preventing yourself developing dementia is thin and relatively unproven. Here is a summary of practical options for you, thoughtfully provided on the subject by the National Health Service. It comes from an organization called NHS Choices – Your Health, Your Choices. I am reproducing it here almost completely, as it reflects much of the content of Chapter 4. However, I must add a warning: the paragraphs on preventing vascular dementia are well founded. As you have read in Chapter 3, those on preventing other types of dementia are less proven. Iris Murdoch was a spectacularly good and prolific writer, and was exceptionally well read, yet she succumbed to devastating dementia. While I am writing this, Terry Pratchett is going through his Alzheimer's stages: his books are testament to the amazing way he used his brain to the full. Nevertheless, what remains of this short chapter is taken entirely from the NHS dementia prevention publication.

Preventing vascular dementia

While it is not possible to prevent all cases of dementia, some measures can help prevent vascular dementia, as well as cardiovascular diseases such as strokes and heart attacks. What is good for your heart is also good for your head.

The best ways to prevent vascular dementia are:

- eat a healthy variety of foods;
- maintain a healthy weight;
- get enough and regular exercise;

- drink alcohol in moderation;
- don't smoke.

Diet

We recommend a low fat and high fibre diet. This includes plenty of fresh fruit, vegetables and wholegrain bread and cereals. Limit your salt intake to no more than 6 grams (around one level teaspoon) a day (in other words, don't use the salt cellar at the table and avoid most processed foods). Too much salt increases blood pressure, which puts you at risk of vascular dementia.

Avoid foods high in saturated fat because this will increase your total blood cholesterol level (about which more later), which also puts you at risk of vascular dementia.

Foods high in saturated fat include:

- meat pies
- sausages and fatty cuts of meat
- butter
- ghee (clarified butter often used in Indian cooking)
- lard
- cream
- hard cheese
- cakes and biscuits
- coconut and palm oil.

Eating foods high in unsaturated fat can decrease cholesterol levels. They include:

- oily fish
- avocados
- nuts and seeds
- sunflower, rapeseed and olive oil.

Weight

Being overweight can increase blood pressure, which increases your risk of vascular dementia. The risk is higher if you are obese. The best way to tackle obesity is to reduce the amount of food you eat and to take regular and enough exercise. Your GP will advise you on the best way to do this.

Exercise

Regular exercise makes your heart and circulation more efficient. It lowers your cholesterol level and keeps the blood pressure at healthy levels, all of which lowers your risk of developing vascular dementia.

For most people we recommend 30 minutes of vigorous exercise a day, at least five days a week. It should be strenuous enough to make your heart beat faster, and you should be slightly out of breath afterwards. Going for a brisk walk or climbing a hill are good examples to follow.

Alcohol

Drinking an excess of alcohol raises your blood pressure and your total blood cholesterol level. Stick to the recommended limits and you should reduce the risk of high blood pressure, cardiovascular disease and vascular dementia. The recommended daily alcohol consumption limit is three to four units for men and two to three units for women. One unit is about half a pint of normal-strength lager, a small glass of wine or a single pub measure of spirits.

Smoking

Smoking causes your arteries to narrow, raising your blood pressure. It is a major risk factor for cardiovascular disease, cancer and vascular dementia. The NHS Smoking Helpline offers advice and encouragement on how to stop smoking, on 0800 022 4332. Visit the NHS Go Smokefree website at <http://smokefree.nhs.uk/>. Your GP and pharmacist will advise on how to stop smoking.

Preventing other types of dementia

There is evidence that rates of dementia are lower in people who remain as mentally and physically active as possible throughout their lives, and have a wide range of different activities and hobbies. Some activities that may reduce your risk of developing dementia include:

- reading
- writing for pleasure
- learning foreign languages
- playing musical instruments
- taking part in adult education courses
- playing tennis
- playing golf
- swimming
- group sports such as bowls
- walking.

There is no evidence that playing brain training computer games reduces the risk of dementia.

That last warning sentence is so definite it is astonishing. Was the writer influenced by his or her annoyance with a teenage son or daughter's computer habits? I wonder. I'm not sure about the evidence for reading, or for golf or simple walking, yet they are promoted in the leaflet. I leave this chapter with a conversation I had with Professor Zaved Khatchaturian, the chairman of the Alzheimer's research group of which I was secretary for a while in the 1990s.

Zaved, originally from Armenia, spoke seven languages. One evening, after a long day discussing research projects, the eight of us were relaxing in an old student pub in Heidelberg. One of the subjects on our agenda that day was the need to keep the brain active – as Hercule Poirot would have said, to exercise the little grey cells. I asked Zaved exactly how much exercise the brain needed to keep itself free from deterioration. I admitted that my own day included trying to complete a difficult cryptic crossword.

He replied, 'In what language do you complete it?'

Naturally I said, 'My own, of course.' I am fluent only in English.

'It isn't enough,' he replied. 'You must learn another language and do your puzzles in it.' Then he laughed, but he meant what he said.

I haven't managed to follow his advice.

6

Dementia provokers 1 – smoking

Over many years as a family doctor I have found that it isn't enough simply to advise people to stop some bad habit, or to help them to start good new habits. I have had to explain, often in great detail, exactly why they should disturb or change their usual routines before they eventually became convinced. It is all very well to say that smoking, drinking, overeating or lounging around in an exercise-free zone is not good for you, but unless I can really convince you that you absolutely need to change to save your life, it won't happen. I can, sadly, put names to dozens of patients whom I tried to help in this way but who failed to adjust, even when their lifestyles were truly life-threatening. I also remember my favourites, the few who did turn themselves around and are still alive today because they were convinced.

So the following chapters are about the habits you must ditch if you are to lower – considerably – your risk of eventual dementia. You may think you know the risks, but that they probably don't apply to you. Please don't make that mistake. They apply to everyone.

Take smoking, for example. Most people know that smoking causes lung problems, such as chronic bronchitis and emphysema or lung cancer. Many understand that it is bad for the heart. Very few, however, realize its role in vascular dementia. Stopping smoking is never one of the steps that people worried about dementia think of taking. In fact, in the past some smokers have maintained that it could even be good for dementia, because they have read that nicotine stimulates the brain cells. They used that as an excuse to carry on. Tragically, it was bosh. Smoking-related dementia is a real and very common disease: it is a major cause of multiple brain infarct dementia, which kills much faster and is at least as traumatic to the victim's family as Alzheimer's disease. So if you smoke, please read the whole of this chapter. If it doesn't make you a non-smoker by its end, you may as well stop reading. You don't need a doctor, but you should make your will.

Why you mustn't smoke

Smoking is a stupid, suicidal habit for anyone, no matter how healthy. It is especially bad for people who may be at risk of dementia and for people who also have diabetes and/or high blood pressure, two of the predisposing conditions for vascular dementia (see Chapter 2). Diabetics and people with high blood pressure (often both come together) are already at higher risk than normal of developing heart disease and strokes, and therefore vascular dementia. If they smoke, they multiply those risks many times over. So what follows is for every smoker, and especially if you also have diabetes and high blood pressure.

How, exactly, does smoking harm you? Tobacco smoke contains carbon monoxide and nicotine. The first poisons the red blood cells, so that they cannot pick up and distribute much-needed oxygen to the organs and tissues, including the heart muscle. Carbon monoxide-affected red cells (in the 20-a-day smoker, nearly 20 per cent of red cells are carrying carbon monoxide instead of oxygen) are also stiffer than normal, so that they can't bend and flex through the smallest blood vessels. The gas also directly poisons the heart muscle, so that it cannot contract properly and efficiently, thereby delivering a 'double whammy' of damage to it.

Nicotine causes small arteries to narrow, so that the blood flow through them slows. It raises blood glucose levels and blood cholesterol levels, thickening the blood and promoting the degenerative process in the artery walls, which is already faster than normal if you have high blood pressure or diabetes. Both nicotine and carbon monoxide encourage the blood to clot, multiplying the risks of coronary thrombosis and a thrombotic stroke.

Add to all this the tars that smoke deposits in the lungs, which further reduce the ability of red cells to pick up oxygen, and the scars and damage to the lungs that always in the end produce chronic bronchitis and sometimes induce cancer, and you have a formula for disaster.

Here are the bald facts about smoking. If they do not convince you to stop, then you may as well give up reading this book, because there is no point in being 'health conscious' if you continue to indulge in tobacco. Its ill effects will counterbalance any good that your doctors can do for you.

- Smoking causes more deaths from heart attacks than from lung cancer and bronchitis.
- People who smoke have two or three times the risk of a fatal heart attack than non-smokers. The risk rises with rising numbers of cigarettes smoked, and is doubled if you are also a diabetic.
- Men under 45 who smoke 25 or more cigarettes a day have a 10–15 times greater chance of death from heart attack than non-smoking men of the same age.
- About 40 per cent of all heavy smokers, even if they do not have diabetes, die before they reach 65. Of those who reach that age, many are disabled by bronchitis, angina, heart failure, leg amputations and dementia, all because they smoked. Diabetes and high blood pressure make all these risks of smoking much greater. Only 10 per cent of smokers survive in reasonable health to the age of 75. Many have dementia by that age, and a sizeable minority of smokers have already died from it before they reached 70. Most non-smokers reach 75 in good health.
- In the UK, 40 per cent of all cancer deaths are from lung cancer, which is very rare in non-smokers. Of 441 British male doctors who died from lung cancer, only seven had never smoked. Only one non-smoker in 60 develops lung cancer: the figure for heavy smokers is one in six!
- Other cancers more common in smokers than in non-smokers include those of the tongue, throat, larynx, pancreas, kidney, bladder and cervix.
- On top of all these lethal effects of tobacco comes the evidence of a 2011 report (in *Archives of Internal Medicine*) on smokers and dementia. Dr Rachel Whitmer followed 21,123 people in their fifties and sixties. The rate of Alzheimer's disease among smokers of more than two packs was 157 per cent higher than in non-

smokers. The corresponding figure for vascular dementia was a whopping 172 per cent.

The very fact that you are reading this book means that you are taking an intelligent interest in your health. So after reading so far, it should be common sense to you not to smoke. Yet it is very difficult to stop, and many people who need an excuse for not stopping put up spurious arguments for their stance. Here are ones that every doctor is tired of hearing, and my replies:

- *My father/grandfather smoked 20 a day and lived till he was 75* Everyone knows someone like that, but they conveniently forget the many others they have known who died long before their time. The chances are that you will be one of them, rather than one of the lucky few.
- *People who don't smoke also have heart attacks* True. There are other causes of heart attacks, but 70 per cent of all people under 65 admitted to coronary care with heart attacks are smokers, as are 91 per cent of people with angina considered for coronary bypass surgery.
- *I believe in moderation in all things, and I only smoke moderately* That's rubbish. We don't accept moderation in mugging, or dangerous driving, or exposure to asbestos (which incidentally causes far fewer deaths from lung cancer than smoking). Younger men who are only moderate smokers have a much higher risk of heart attack than non-smoking men of the same age. The figures are even worse for women with diabetes, who have a higher risk of heart attack than non-diabetic men of the same age.
- *I can cut down on cigarettes, but I can't stop* It won't do you much good if you do. People who cut down usually inhale more from each cigarette and leave a smaller butt, so that they end up with the same blood levels of nicotine and carbon monoxide. You must stop completely.
- *I'm just as likely to be run over in the road as to die from my smoking* In the UK about 15 people die on the roads each day. This contrasts with 100 deaths a day from lung cancer, 100 from chronic

bronchitis and 100 from heart attacks, almost all of which are due to smoking. The number of cases of dementia in smokers isn't known precisely, because one of these three causes is usually on the death certificates. Very many of such certificates don't mention the fact that there has also been accompanying dementia in the smokers who have fortuitously survived long enough to develop it. Of every 1,000 young men who smoke, on average one will be murdered, six will die on the roads, and 250 will die from their smoking habit. Increase those numbers for men and women with diabetes and/or high blood pressure.

- *I have to die from something* In my experience this is always said by someone in good health. They no longer say it after their heart attack or stroke, or after they have coughed up blood. Of course, they can't say it if they have vascular dementia.
- *I don't want to be old, anyway* We define 'old' differently as we grow older. Most of us would like to live a long time, without the inconvenience of being old. If we take care of ourselves on the way to becoming old, we have at least laid the foundations for enjoying our old age. That's one of the reasons that you are reading this book. One way to do that is to fend off dementia. Stopping smoking will help to do that.
- *I'd rather die of a heart attack than something else* Most of us would like a fast, sudden death, but many heart attack victims leave a grieving partner in their early fifties to face thirty years of loneliness. And many dementia victims cause years of anguish for their families and friends. Is that really what you wish?
- *Stress, not smoking, is the main cause of heart attacks* Not true. Stress is very difficult to measure and it is very difficult to relate it to heart attack rates. In any case, you have to cope with stress, whether you smoke or not. Smoking is an extra burden that can never help, and it does not relieve stress. It isn't burning the candle at both ends that causes harm but burning the cigarette at one end. As an aside, long-term stress, which is increased – not decreased – by smoking, also strongly contributes to dementia.
- *I'll stop when I start to feel ill* That would be fine if the first sign of illness were not a full-blown heart attack from which more than

a third die in the first four hours. It's too late to stop then. If your illness is vascular dementia you will no longer be able to make the decision to stop, so it will continue to progress.

- *I'll put on weight if I stop smoking* You probably will, because your appetite will return and you will be able to taste food again, but the benefits of stopping smoking far outweigh the few extra pounds you may put on.

- *I enjoy smoking and don't want to give it up* Is that really true? Is that not just an excuse because you can't stop? Ask yourself what your real pleasure is in smoking, and try to be honest with the answer.

- *Cigarettes settle my nerves. If I stopped I'd have to take a tranquillizer* Smoking is a prop, like a baby's dummy, but it solves nothing. It doesn't remove any causes of stress, and only makes things worse because it adds a promoter of bad health. And when you start to have symptoms, like the regular morning cough, it only makes you worry more. Of course, if it leads to dementia you will forget what you are worrying about, but that doesn't make up for the disaster it causes to you and your family.

- *I'll change to a pipe or cigar – they are safer* Lifelong pipe and cigar smokers are less prone than cigarette smokers to heart attacks, but have five times the risk of lung cancer and ten times the risk of chronic bronchitis compared with non-smokers. Cigarette smokers who switch to pipes or cigars continue to be at high risk of heart attack, probably because they inhale.

- *I've been smoking for 30 years – it's too late to stop now* It's not too late whenever you stop. The risk of sudden death from a first heart attack falls away very quickly after stopping, even after a lifetime of smoking. If you stop after surviving a heart attack then you halve the risk of a second. It takes longer to reduce your risk of lung cancer, but it falls by 80 per cent over the next 15 years, no matter how long you have been a smoker.

- *I wish I could stop. I've tried everything, but nothing has worked* Stopping smoking isn't easy unless you really want to do it. You have to make the effort yourself, rather than think that someone else can do it for you. So you must be motivated. If the next few pages do not motivate you, then nothing will.

How to stop smoking

You must find the right reason for yourself to stop. For someone worried about dementia you should convince yourself that you have a much better chance of remaining healthy into your old age. But there are plenty of other reasons.

For teenagers and young adults (hopefully some are reading this), who see middle age and sickness as remote possibilities and who see smoking as exciting and dangerous, the best attacks on smoking are the way it makes them look and smell. You can also add the environmental pollution of cigarette ends and the way big business exploits less affluent nations, keeping their populations in poverty while they make huge profits from putting land that should be growing food under tobacco cultivation. Pakistan uses 120,000 acres, and Brazil half a million acres, of their richest agricultural land to grow tobacco. And as the multinationals are now promoting their product very heavily to poorer countries, no teenager who smokes can claim to be really concerned about the health of the Global South. This is often as persuasive an argument in encouraging a teenager to stop (or not to start) as any about health or looks.

For some older women, the key may be looks. Smoking ages people prematurely, causing wrinkles and giving a pale, pasty complexion. Women smokers experience the menopause at an earlier age, even in their mid-thirties, which can destroy the plans of businesswomen to have their families after a shot at a career.

For men and other women the prime motivation is better health. The statistics for non-diabetic men and women in their sixties who smoke are frightening enough, without bringing in the possibility of dementia to further worsen them. More than a third of smoking men fail to reach pension age – add many more to that figure if they also have diabetes of either type or high blood pressure.

Let us assume you are now fully motivated. How do you stop? It is easy. You become a non-smoker, as if you have never smoked. You throw away all your cigarettes and decide never to buy or accept another one. Announce the fact to all your friends, who will usually support you, and that's that. Most people find that they don't have true withdrawal symptoms, provided they are happy to stop. A few become agitated, irritable, nervous and can't sleep at night. But people who have had to stop for medical reasons – say, because they have been admitted to coronary care – hardly ever have withdrawal symptoms.

That strongly suggests that such symptoms are psychological rather than physical. If you can last a week or two without a smoke, you will probably never light up again. The desire to smoke will disappear as the levels of carbon monoxide, nicotine and tarry chemicals in your lungs, blood, brain and other organs gradually subside.

If you must stop gradually, plan ahead. Write out a diary of the cigarettes you will have, leaving out one or two each succeeding day, and stick to it. Carry nicotine chewing gum or get a patch if you must, but remember that the nicotine is still harmful. Don't look on it as a long-term alternative to a smoke. If you are having real difficulty stopping, ask your doctor for a prescription of Zyban. You may be offered a two-month course of the drug. It helps, but is by no means infallible. Most health centres now offer a smoking cessation clinic. Ask your doctor about it. There you will be sympathetically supported as you stop and are helped to keep smoke-free. Our local clinic has a very high success rate, mainly because of the enthusiasm of the staff (several of whom are ex-smokers).

If you do use aids to stop (others include acupuncture and hypnosis), remember they have no magical properties. They are a crutch to lean on while you make the determined effort to stop altogether. They cannot help if your will to stop is weak.

Recognize, too, that stopping smoking is not an end in itself. It is only part of your new way of life, which includes your new way of eating and exercise and your new attitude to your future health. And you owe it not only to yourself but also to your partner, family and friends, because it will help to give them a healthier you for, hopefully, years to come. You are not on your own. More than a million Britons have stopped smoking each year for the last fifteen years. Only one in four adults now smokes (fewer than one in 40 doctors do so). By stopping you are joining the sensible majority.

7

Dementia provokers 2 – alcohol

The one social habit that has changed the most over the last few decades is our attitude to alcohol. The drinking laws have become much more liberal, and alcoholic drinks have become much more freely available, relatively cheaper and much stronger than they were as recently as the 1980s. Teenagers and young adults seem to have much more money to spend on alcoholic drinks, and varieties of alcoholic drinks such as alcopops have been specially developed for them. They have taken to them like ducks to water – but with much less desirable results.

The biggest change has been in young women. They have taken to the new culture of weekend boozing in city centres as if their lives depended on it: which, sadly, they do. As a young doctor I was taught that liver and brain disease due to alcohol rarely developed in women under the age of 50, and that even in older women they were far less common than in men of the same age. In my student days the ratio of men to women with serious chronic alcohol-induced disease was 20 to one.

Today, from the late twenties onwards, women are matching men in their alcohol-related illness rates. Sadly, many of them have never realized that they were drinking too much. Last summer I had to tell a 37-year-old businesswoman that her liver was so affected by alcoholic cirrhosis that she needed a transplant, but that she would not be accepted for it unless she managed to last three months without drinking at all.

She was astonished: she had never been the worse for her drinking, she explained. She and her husband, she admitted, drank two or three glasses of wine each evening, and she also had one at occasional lunchtime business meetings. We counted up her alcohol score. She used 250 ml glasses, and drank wine at around 12 to 13 per cent proof. This amounted to five units a day, or 35 units a week

– far above the 14 accepted as the upper limit for women before liver and brain damage starts to become evident.

Her husband had asked her to see me. She had lost weight, was thin, with a slight yellow tinge to the whites of her eyes. When she stretched out her hands and a thin paper sheet was placed over her fingers, the paper shook. Asked to flex back her hands to make an angle with her wrists, she couldn't maintain that position without the palms jerking forward every few seconds – a classical sign of liver disease we call 'liver flap'. Her palms were red, rather than pink. She had dozens of spider naevi (tiny red spots from which spidery 'legs' extended) over her chest and body.

All these were classical signs of severe liver disease, and the diagnosis was confirmed by blood tests, particularly one called gammaGT, which showed an exceptionally high reading.

All this was worrying enough, but what worried me even more was that, during our meeting, she repeated herself several times. A few tactful questions revealed that she was not as up to date with current events as she, as an astute businesswoman, should have been. I wondered if she had a condition called Korsakoff's syndrome, in which the alcohol-damaged brain loses its short-term memory. A simple test of memory confirmed it.

All I could do initially was to refer her to our local liver specialist and to counsel her against her drinking. She wouldn't accept that she had been drinking too much until I showed her the results of her tests a few days later. Six months further on, she had her transplant and she is now, a year later, the picture of health. She has a healthy liver and has forsworn alcohol. Sadly, however, her brain damage remains and will probably be permanent. She has lost her job and is finding it difficult to adjust to her new circumstances. Luckily her husband is supporting her.

This story was highly unusual in the 1980s; now, tragically, it is commonplace.

Alcohol and smoking produce different types of dementia. Smokers have multi-infarct disease, mainly because of all the properties of tobacco smoke, described in the previous chapter, that promote blood clotting and arterial wall degeneration. Heavy drinkers directly poison their liver and brain cells. In contrast to what happens in smokers, their blood clots less easily than normal, mainly because their poisoned livers can't produce the proteins involved in the complex chain of events that lead to clotting, or thrombosis. Instead, alcohol abuse leads to bleeding from the brain blood vessels, leading to 'haemorrhagic' stroke, the immediate and long-term (if the patient survives) consequences of which are usually more serious than the 'thrombotic' kind linked to smoking.

Just as devastating is alcohol's direct effect on brain cells: in larger than minimal doses alcohol is a direct nerve cell poison. When it is taken over months and years the brain cells die off, in a process named alcoholic encephalopathy, and the result, if the habit is not given up in its early years, is irreversible dementia.

What are safe limits?

Much of the work done on exactly how much we can safely drink before damaging ourselves was done by Professor Roger Williams' team at King's College Hospital, London. Professor Williams was a liver specialist, not a psychiatrist, so he approached the problem from physical, medical and pathological points of view rather than a more psychological one, and his results and conclusions reflected these interests. Based on his work we now have very specific advice to give to all social drinkers. If you wish to remain reasonably compos mentis and to avoid alcohol-linked dementia, please follow it.

You could be forgiven for being confused about the various messages we doctors have been promoting about alcohol. In the early 1990s the idea of 'safe' amounts of alcohol was promoted, so that it became acceptable for men to drink 21 and women to drink 14 units a week without doing themselves any long-term harm. That came to be seen as meaning that drinking up to that amount of alcohol was actually good for you – not the same message at all.

Then the red wine message hit the lay press. It came from a study by Professor Jean-Marc Orgogozo and his team at Bordeaux University. I met Professor Orgogozo at the meeting at which he presented his findings, and liked him a lot. He is a good scientist and is not funded by any special interest, such as the wine-makers.

He started his research with the idea that regular drinking of red wine from a very early age, as happens in his region, might be harmful, so he followed drinkers and non-drinkers for many years, noting what they died from and at what age. He was astonished to find that the wine-drinkers outlived the non-drinkers by several years, and the difference persisted when he removed all the other possible influences that might have prolonged their lives (or shortened the non-drinkers' lives).

Clearly something in the red wine helped to protect drinkers from heart attacks and strokes. Was it the alcohol or a particular property of the wine unrelated to it? The academic argument continued: well-respected researchers in Edinburgh and in Munich reported similar saving of lives by moderate drinking of whisky or beer. The figures were supported by surveys of millions of deaths reported to life assurance companies, which proved that lifelong teetotallers tend to die a year or two before moderate drinkers.

So is a little alcohol each day a good thing for you, if you think you may be prone to dementia? Much depends on what you define as a little, and whether you can keep it to a little. The standard advice became that women should drink no more than two to three units of alcohol a day, while men were allowed three to four. A unit meant a single measure of spirits (a 'half' in Scotland), a standard glass of wine, a small glass of fortified wine like sherry or port, or a half-pint (250 ml) of beer – even less than that if it is a strong beer.

The message certainly got home to the public. It may just have been a coincidence, but when the message about the health benefits of wine reached the public, the amounts drunk nationwide ballooned. Of course, this was a time when we became much more affluent, the price of alcohol dropped against the rate of inflation, and young adults had much more money in their pockets. No single change in society was to blame, but many more people than ever before drank much more alcohol than ever before.

The drinks changed, too. Today's wines are much stronger, at 12 to 13 per cent proof, than the wines we drank only a few years ago (at around 8 to 10 per cent proof). And our wine glasses, which used to contain 125 ml, now hold 250 ml. As the original 'unit' was based on the 125 ml glass at 8 per cent proof, our habit of swallowing 250 ml of 13 per cent wine gives us three units per glass. One glass per day is more than enough for a woman and is the recommended upper dose for a man! How many people stick to a single glass per day? And how many give their livers and brains a non-alcoholic rest on three days every week? In my experience as a GP, very few. That three-day rest from alcohol has also turned out to be important: the brain and liver perform better if we abstain on a few days a week. I don't have proof that doing so might help prevent dementia, but it seems likely.

However, abstaining for weekdays and bingeing at weekends is not an answer. People who get smashed at weekends are probably doing themselves more harm than the steady daily drinker of a glass or two.

There is an extra risk for the weekend binger. They often fall over! And unlike cyclists and motorcyclists, they don't wear protective headgear. Repeated head injuries are a major cause of later dementia. It is enough for the moment to state that with each such 'accident' the combination of alcohol and brain trauma makes eventual dementia more certain. The type of dementia tends to be a mixed one, with multiple small brain bruises and tears destroying for good the brain tissues around them, and the accumulation of episodes of alcohol poisoning what is left. So alcohol abusers (and remember the patient with whom I began this chapter – you don't have to drink much to become an abuser) develop an illness that combines the characteristics of Alzheimer's and multi-infarct disease. It is a very heavy price to pay for their drinking habits.

If you have diabetes – alcohol and diabetes don't go together

If you happen also to have diabetes, the message about alcohol and dementia becomes even more strict. Keeping good control over your diabetes is incompatible with excess alcohol, and there is a strong link between a lifetime of poor diabetes control and eventual dementia. So I make no apology for including a little about diabetes and alcohol here.

To start with, alcohol is a high source of calories (1 gram gives you 7 calories), so you must take that into account when you are giving yourself your insulin. Second, too much alcohol drunk over even a moderate period can start to harm your liver, brain and peripheral nerves – the nerves running between your limbs and spinal cord that detect sensations (pain, touch, heat, cold, vibration, position sense) and initiate muscle action. If you regularly overdo your alcohol intake you are inviting liver, brain and nerve disease, and once they have been established they are hard to reverse.

If you already have signs of peripheral neuropathy (your specialist will, hopefully, already have done the necessary tests for it) even moderate amounts of alcohol can make it worse. A relatively minor loss of sensation in the fingers and toes can develop into constant pins and needles, numbness and inability to tell when water is scalding hot or freezing cold. And as peripheral nerves run to and from the genital area, one sign of diabetic neuropathy is impotence. Alcohol ruins the performance even of non-diabetics (read the gatekeeper scene in *Macbeth*): if you have Type 1 diabetes the combination of alcohol and neuropathy can leave you impotent long after the hangover has gone.

So it is wise for all Type 1 diabetics to keep their alcohol intake down to the minimum, say one or two units a day at most, and have several days a week alcohol-free. If you already have neuropathy, seriously consider whether you can do without alcohol altogether.

Whether or not you have diabetes, the next piece of advice on alcohol is relevant to you. Don't drink on an empty stomach. Alcohol on an empty stomach can drive your blood glucose level down – into the 'hypo' region if you are diabetic. Repeated 'hypos' (low blood-glucose episodes) in diabetes can lead to permanent brain injury and dementia, so they need to be avoided. Drinking so much that you become semi-conscious has a similar effect even if you are not diabetic. So if you must have a pre-meal drink, then have a starch-rich snack with it, such as a sandwich. That's important, too, at bedtime, if you like a small 'nightcap'. Don't have the drink on its own – have a savoury biscuit or a small sandwich with it. Otherwise you may have a hypo during the night, with its accompanying nightmares, and restlessness and headache in the morning. In countries like Italy and France, people enjoy their alcohol as an accompaniment to their food. They rarely drink simply to get drunk, in a drinks-only atmosphere. It is the civilized way to enjoy alcohol, and it also prevents them (usually!) from drinking too much at one time. They take hours over their meals and their drinks. And they seem to have a more enjoyable old age.

Alcohol and high blood pressure

One unfortunate consequence of the message coming from the studies by Professor Orgogozo and his colleagues, that 'a little drink will do you good', is that for many people it was wrong. For some years we believed that drinking a little alcohol a day lowered blood pressure, by opening up the small arteries (that's why we flush when we drink) and increasing blood flow to the brain and heart. By doing so, it was argued, we could protect ourselves against heart attacks. So doctors even began to recommend it to people at risk of heart disease and strokes, and even to people who were already known to have heart problems.

Enter Dr Gareth Beevers, of Birmingham's City (Dudley Road) Hospital. An internationally renowned specialist in high blood pressure, he showed from his database of thousands of patients with high blood pressure that blood pressure rises steeply with the amount of alcohol drunk. There was no blip in the straight line upwards from the smallest amount of alcohol to the highest: the more we drink, the higher is our blood pressure.

His conclusion was that if you have a high blood pressure problem, then drinking even the smallest amount of alcohol will make it worse. That is bad for the heart and brain, in that it makes heart attacks and strokes much more likely. Just as important, a constantly higher blood pressure than you need for good health predisposes to multi-infarct dementia. So if you have high blood pressure, be very careful about the amount you drink regularly: consult your doctor about how much you can drink safely. A diary of daily blood pressure measurements plotted against your alcohol consumption should convince you. Your ration is likely to be considerably less than three units a day.

Why, if you have raised blood pressure, you should do all you can to bring it down into the normal levels is the subject, therefore, of the next chapter.

8

Dementia provokers 3 –
high blood pressure

James Watson is 60. He took early retirement this year, while he was 'still
healthy enough to enjoy it'. He is physically and mentally active, takes a
pride in his garden and can still do *The Times* crossword every day. He has
a little arthritis, so he can't bend as well as he used to, but he compen-
sates for that by swimming three or four times a week and walking briskly
for two or three miles every day. In short, he is the ideal patient – one
who hardly ever sees his doctor, except for an occasional repeat prescription for a non-steroidal anti-inflammatory drug (NSAID).

So why am I worried about him? At his annual health check his blood
pressure turned out to be 170/85 mmHg (millimetres of mercury –
the standard way we measure blood pressure). This is definitely too
high, but does he need treatment for it when he has absolutely no
symptoms?

Following the principle of the previous two chapters, here is an
explanation of normal and high blood pressure. It sets out precisely
why you should take your blood pressure readings seriously if you
wish to help yourself avoid dementia.

Blood pressure – what you need to know

Normal blood vessels, and in particular the arteries that carry blood
from your heart to your organs and tissues, are smooth-lined tubes
through which the blood flows without hindrance or eddy cur-
rents, like the water supply to your house. Their walls are elastic, so
that they expand to cope with extra flow and relax when you rest.
They are also muscular, so that they can push the blood onwards in
concert with the heartbeat and pulse.

There are two components of the blood pressure, the 'systolic' pressure and the 'diastolic' pressure. The first is the pressure exerted on the blood by the beat of the heart. When the lower chambers of the heart, the ventricles, contract, they push the blood into the arteries, and the pressure of that 'push' (medically the term is 'systole') is the systolic pressure. When the ventricles relax and expand with the flow of blood into them from the atria (the two upper chambers) above them, this is 'diastole'. In diastole, the valves leading from the ventricles into the arteries close off to prevent the blood from flowing back into the heart from the arteries, and the forward pressure of the blood is maintained by the tension in the artery walls – this is the diastolic pressure.

So when we take the blood pressure we note it down as two figures – the systolic and diastolic pressures. They are measured in millimetres of mercury (mmHg) and separated by a forward slash. So a person with a systolic pressure of 120 mmHg and a diastolic pressure of 80 mmHg will be noted as having a blood pressure of 120/80 (the systolic pressure is always higher than the diastolic). James's pressure of 170/85 is too high and puts him at risk.

Normally, your blood pressure remains steady through quite a narrow range. When you exercise or are under stress it goes up, but when you lie back, rest and relax, it should fall again. Only when the blood pressure remains well above normal when you are in a relaxed physical and mental state are you considered to have high blood pressure, or 'hypertension'.

If your blood pressure remains in the normal range throughout your life, then your arteries tend to remain healthy, with smooth surfaces over which the blood can flow without turbulence. If the blood pressure rises, the structure of the arterial walls has to change to cope with the extra strain on them. They become more muscular, they lose some of their elasticity and, in the process of thickening, their diameter narrows, so that there is less room in which the blood can flow. Think of gripping a hosepipe hard and feeling the extra pressure under which the water is flowing, and you will get the idea.

If the arteries become narrower, the heart needs to pump harder to force the blood through them, and that raises the systolic pressure. But the narrowing has another effect, too. If it is due to muscle thickening, then the smaller arteries exert more force on their contents, and this explains the rise in diastolic pressure. If the high blood pressure persists, then a vicious circle starts, with the heart beating ever harder and the arteries responding with more thickening, so that the systolic, then the diastolic, pressure continues to rise.

In normal health, your kidneys are essential to the control of your blood pressure. When the blood pressure falls, as in sleep, the kidneys secrete a substance called renin into the bloodstream. In the kidneys are cells that monitor the pressure of the blood flowing through their arteries: their automatic reaction to lowered blood pressure is to produce renin. When the renin reaches the bloodstream it sets off a chain of chemical reactions, the final link in which is another chemical called angiotensin. The effect of angiotensin on the small blood vessels in the limbs is to make them narrow (a process we call 'vasoconstriction'). In the normal state, with normal kidneys and normal blood pressure, just enough angiotensin is formed from renin to bring a low blood pressure into the normal range.

Sadly, not everyone's kidneys are completely efficient. They may produce more renin than normal (probably in an effort to increase poor blood flow through the glomeruli, the tiny units within the kidney where blood is cleaned). The blood pressure rises constantly, and another vicious circle starts. The more renin the kidney produces, the higher is the blood pressure, and the higher the blood pressure the more damage it wreaks on the delicate blood vessels in the kidneys. The more damaged the kidney becomes, the more renin it produces, and the circle is cranked up another notch.

Knowledge of this biochemical mechanism has led to the development of drugs that interrupt this circle. Drugs called angiotensin-converting enzyme inhibitors (ACE inhibitors) or angiotensin II blockers (ATII blockers) prevent the formation of angiotensin by renin. They have the double benefit of lowering blood pressure and protecting the kidneys from further damage. They and other drugs to control high blood pressure are described on pp. 78–9.

Renin has yet another effect. It also reaches the adrenal glands, which lie across the upper surface of the kidneys. They respond to the hormone by producing another hormone, aldosterone, which causes the kidneys to retain extra water and sodium. That increases your whole body volume, and that raises the blood pressure further. We can use 'aldosterone antagonists' to block this action, too.

As if three mechanisms to push up the blood pressure weren't enough, there is a fourth one. All arteries are controlled by the 'sympathetic nervous system', a network of nerves that, when stimulated, cause the muscles in artery walls to contract. That causes the arteries to narrow, just like that grip around a hosepipe mentioned earlier. Some people have arteries that overreact to the sympathetic 'message'. For them, the choice of drug could well be a sympathetic blocker drug – known to doctors as 'alpha-blockers' or 'beta-blockers'.

By now you have begun to understand how complex the choice of drugs for high blood pressure can be, and why your doctors have a set of guidelines, worked out by the country's experts, that they follow for prescribing them.

To summarize: if you know you have high blood pressure, it is vital that you get it under control so that it lies within the normal range for blood pressure in the population. If you wish to avoid multi-infarct dementia or dementia following a stroke, then you must do your best to know what your blood pressure is and how to keep it as low as possible. The lower your blood pressure is, within the normal range, the better are your prospects of preventing maxi- or mini-strokes, and therefore of dementia.

Your doctor will have several ways of achieving this, with drugs such as diuretics, ACE inhibitors or ATII blockers, aldosterone inhibitors, beta-blockers and perhaps other drugs. Your contribution to this care is to take your chosen treatment assiduously, treating it with the same importance as someone with diabetes would insulin.

If you would like to know more about high blood pressure and how you and your medical team can work together to control it, please read *Living with High Blood Pressure*, another of my Sheldon Press books.

I wish I could write that this is all you need to know about your risks from hypertension, but it isn't. There is a companion problem to high blood pressure that you also need to know all about if you are to take best care of your kidneys, and that is atheroma. You must fight it with just as much will as you tackle hypertension.

Atheroma – your heart and your brain

When we are children the inner linings of our heart and arteries – the surfaces that are in contact with our blood – are smooth and their walls muscular and elastic. The blood flows remarkably smoothly, without any turbulence, through them.

Sadly, as we grow older this changes. Fatty deposits start to be laid down in the blood-vessel walls. The more fat our bloodstream carries around with it, the more fatty deposits there are. The process starts early. US doctors examining the bodies of young soldiers killed in the Korean War were astonished by the extent of the fatty degeneration in their aortas – the main artery leaving the heart to supply the head, chest, abdomen and limbs. There were even fatty streaks in the young men's coronary arteries, which supply the heart muscle itself. These findings led to the first US efforts to prevent heart disease.

This laying-down of fats in the walls of arteries has a name – atheroma. It is derived from the ancient Greek word for porridge, because the deposits had the look and consistency of blobs of porridge. It's important to remember that this is nothing to do with 'hardening of the arteries', in which the arteries stiffen as the elastic cells in the walls become more fibrous. That is a natural development of old age and quite a separate development from atheroma.

Deposits – or, to use the medical name, 'plaques' – of atheroma appear in the arteries from childhood onwards. Their numbers and size are closely related to two properties of the circulation: the pressure within it and the level of fats (or 'lipids') in the blood. The best-known fat is cholesterol, and it can't have escaped you, unless you have been living on a desert island alone and without a radio for the last thirty years, that the higher your cholesterol level, the higher your chances are of a heart attack or stroke. It also can't have escaped you that living a lifestyle that lowers your cholesterol, along with taking cholesterol-lowering drugs, will help you avoid or at least postpone such catastrophes.

What has this to do with preventing dementia? Actually, quite a lot, although the experts did debate the issue for years before they came to solid conclusions about the links between hypertension, atheroma and a raised risk of heart attack or stroke.

The medical literature on the link goes back to 1983, when John C. Van Stone, Professor of Medicine of the University of Missouri in Columbia, Missouri, wrote his book *Dialysis and the Treatment of Renal Insufficiency*. Commenting on the increase in deaths due to heart attacks and strokes in dialysis patients, he was sure that the fundamental problem was their hypertension. Their constant exposure to high blood pressure, he wrote, was the main reason for the 'accelerated atheroma' that underlay their sudden deaths. Only when there was a history of hypertension in a patient was there also evidence of atheroma severe enough to shorten their lives. Without it, kidney patients with normal blood pressure were no more at risk of heart attack or stroke than people of the same age and gender without kidney disease. That book was seminal to our understanding now of the relationship between high blood pressure and atheroma, and therefore of strokes and stroke-linked dementia. Although Professor Van Stone was writing about his speciality, serious kidney disease, his conclusions are relevant to everyone from early adulthood onwards.

Professor Van Stone was not seeing patients with milder kidney disease – people who would never have to come to him for dialysis or transplant. Today, if you have been told you have moderate renal failure, you will be advised very firmly that your main future health problem will not lie in your kidney failure, but in your higher than average risk of heart attack and stroke. Equally firmly, you will be told that these have three main causes – hypertension, a high blood cholesterol level and smoking.

Why has there been such a change? Thirty years ago, when Professor Van Stone was writing, he (and all other doctors practising at the time) didn't know the true extent of mild and moderate kidney disease in the population. More important, we didn't know its relevance to atheroma and consequently to heart attacks and strokes. What brought about the change was our routine use of more sophisticated tests and measurements to find out who, among our 'healthy' patients, actually had a time-bomb ticking in their kidneys. Only when we began to use these tests did we realize their significance. Many people have been found to have moderate kidney disease because they have atheroma. It is the fatty degeneration in their arteries that is the main cause of their poor kidney function, and it is a 'red flag' indicating that they have to try to reverse it. This is clearly a separate aim: in addition to lowering their blood pressure, they must also attend to their cholesterol level.

You may not think this is relevant to you: after all, you don't have moderate kidney disease, do you? You may be surprised. When we family doctors in Scotland started routine testing for it (using a blood test called the 'estimated glomerular filtration rate' or eGFR) among our healthy population, we found that a massive one in ten of our patients over 50 years old have it. For the vast majority of them their result came as a severe shock – because they had only been to the doctor for a routine health check. It was natural for them, on hearing that they had chronic kidney disease, to fear that they would end up in the dialysis or transplant clinic.

In fact, fewer than one in 100 of such people do find themselves in end-stage kidney failure. What they do face, however, is a higher than average risk of strokes and heart attacks, and in particular multiple small strokes, leading to probable dementia.

Your personal plumbing

Look upon your circulation as a closed, flexible, elastic tube with a pump (your heart) and auxiliary pumping stations (the muscles in the walls of your arteries) along the way. Imagine such a system as heating your house. If the water pressure is too high, the tubing may crack under the strain and burst. If the lining of the tubing is furred up with deposits of material (say, lime-scale in a hard-water area) then the water can't flow through it, and without a plumber to remove the scale the flow will eventually stop. If the boiler has to work too hard to pump the water through the tubing, it will burst. Or if the pump is neglected and corrodes, it will break down.

Of course, the analogies are simplistic, but they do bear some thought. High water pressure equates to high blood pressure. The lime-scale idea isn't too different from deposits of calcium or cholesterol in the lining of arteries in the heart, brain and kidneys – and it has the same effect of reducing the flow. It is a good model for what happens in strokes, heart attacks and multi-infarct dementia. And if you neglect your 'pump', you are looking forward to heart failure.

Let's turn back from domestic piping to humans. The blood pressure risk is at the basis of cardiovascular disease, but along with it you need to tackle your high cholesterol (your plaques of atheroma) and, of course, if you indulge, your smoking. Any one of these risks is bad enough: if you have two, then it is serious. If you admit to all three, and don't want to change, then you should be starting to think of putting your affairs in order. Other people can't help you unless you are determined to help yourself.

Managing your blood pressure

Let me ask you the question James Watson, with his pressure of 170/85, asked me. Why treat my high blood pressure at all? This is a perfectly reasonable question, especially if, when you didn't know you had it, you felt perfectly well. And then you didn't feel so well once you started treatment. That's the case for many people who are found, incidentally, to have high blood pressure.

We doctors are always hearing four arguments against treating high blood pressure. They are:

1 I felt well when I had the high blood pressure, but the drugs you give me have unpleasant side effects. Why should I take a drug that makes me feel worse?
2 I've heard that lots of people with high blood pressure live normally into old age with no problems, when the statistics suggest that they should have died years before. Why couldn't I be in that group?
3 You can't prove to me that, as an individual, using drugs to keep my blood pressure low will prolong my life. So why should I take them?
4 Treating high blood pressure involves me not only taking drugs but also changing almost all aspects of my life. Is the change worth the bother?

Our best way to answer these questions is to tell you about the risks you run if we don't control your blood pressure. There are two kinds of evidence for them – what happens to individuals with hypertension as they grow older, and the statistics for deaths from hypertension, including from life assurance companies. They base their premium rates on blood pressure measurements: their figures are carefully calculated and are the most accurate measure of the extent to which hypertension shortens life.

However, my feelings on hypertension as a doctor are based on my experiences with patients in the days before we had really effective treatments for it. In my medical student days there were always patients suffering from the last stages of high blood pressure, many of them still young. Two of them I still remember well. One was a schoolteacher, aged 40, with a loving family and everything to live for, who died of a heart attack after a series of strokes. The other was a young woman who developed severe hypertension in her first pregnancy and two years later died of kidney failure.

Today, neither would have died. The schoolteacher would have responded well to today's drugs and could have expected to live into a normal old age. The young mother would have had her pregnancy high blood pressure managed efficiently and would not have gone on into kidney failure. Until the 1970s, high blood pressure often ended up as a condition called 'malignant hypertension' with the sufferer going blind, suffering minor strokes and dying from kidney failure because of the damage the extreme pressure did to the delicate circulation in his or her nephrons. Once you developed malignant hypertension you didn't survive a year, despite the best of treatment.

Doctors who have qualified since the 1970s have never seen a full-blown case of malignant hypertension, purely because we now have powerful and highly effective antihypertensive drugs. We not only know that they work, we also know how they work and on which part of the body's pressure-regulating system they act. This is a huge advantage, especially for high blood pressure linked to kidney disease.

This, for me, is the best argument for active treatment of all cases of hypertension – even when it is classified as 'moderate' or 'mild'. You may find it inconvenient, but it is far better than the alternative.

How high blood pressure harms you

Just to hammer an extra nail in the coffin of untreated high blood pressure, and for you to read when you think you might stop your treatment, I have outlined here how your circulation reacts to untreated high blood pressure.

The arteries

Your blood vessels take the main brunt of the constantly high pressure, and they have to change to cope with it. Their walls thicken to withstand the extra force applied to them. Their inner linings, normally smooth to allow fast flow of the blood inside them, become roughened, thus narrowing the diameter of the channel through which the blood has to flow.

In these narrowed, roughened, thickened arteries the blood flow becomes sluggish. The blood becomes stickier as it is pushed by the pressure through the narrowed vessels, and tends to clot more easily than usual. The scene is set for a thrombosis: a lump of solid clotted blood, attached to the roughened artery wall, closes it off completely. If it is in a coronary artery – one that supplies the heart – you will have a heart attack. If it is in a cerebral artery, serving the brain, you will have a stroke.

The high pressure may rupture a weakened artery in the brain so that blood escapes into the brain substance. This 'cerebral haemorrhage' leaves you with a severe stroke, with serious after-effects such as paralysis and loss of feeling, and it may be fatal.

The heart

Your heart, too, can be damaged by longstanding untreated high blood pressure. In the beginning it copes with the strain of maintaining the high pressure by increasing its muscle bulk, enlarging so that it can pump harder. Eventually it can't enlarge more without losing efficiency. The continuing high pressure expands and thins it, so that it becomes like an overblown balloon.

At this stage the pump starts to fail. The heart can no longer drive the volume of fluid in the circulation around the body, and some of it begins to accumulate in tissues such as the legs and the lungs.

The main symptoms are breathlessness on the least exertion and swollen feet and ankles. If the swelling is pressed with a finger a small pit-like depression is left in the waterlogged flesh.

This is 'congestive heart failure' or CHF. In the past it was a common way for people with high blood pressure to die. Happily, it is not so today.

The kidneys

Constant high blood pressure causes the small arteries in the kidneys to thicken in exactly the same way as the arteries in the heart and brain. It is especially serious for the kidneys, as the result is not simply a matter of poor circulation. The effect is to make the damaged organs even less able to perform their function of filtering the blood and producing urine.

In the past we didn't have effective antihypertensive drugs, and we couldn't tell, when we were dealing with people in the last stages of kidney failure, whether the initial illness had been kidney disease that had produced high blood pressure, or high blood pressure that had produced kidney disease. Their final clinical pictures were identical. It is many years, happily, since a patient in the practices in which I work today had such uncontrollable hypertension that it led to kidney failure. This is a huge credit to the benefits of modern drugs and to the way today's doctors manage all our patients with high blood pressure, regardless of its origin. It is also a credit to the patients whom we treat, and who co-operate in such a willing way with our advice.

The proof that lowering blood pressure into the normal range saves lives came as long ago as 1982, with the results of two massive trials in Australia and the USA. They followed more than 10,000 mildly hypertensive men and women in the two countries. The Australians divided 3,420 subjects, all with only mildly raised blood pressure, into two groups with equal numbers. One group was given active drugs to bring blood pressure into the normal range, while the other was given placebo. Over the following five years there were four deaths in the 'active' group and 13 in the placebo group – a difference that could not have been expected by chance. Many more people in the placebo group than in the active group also had non-fatal heart attacks and strokes. As the active group had on average a diastolic blood pressure around 5 to 7 mmHg lower than that in the placebo group, it was reasonable to conclude that the lower pressure was the direct cause of the lower death and illness rates.

In the US trial half of the 7,800 patients were treated intensively by the research doctors themselves, and half were referred back to their GPs for routine blood pressure follow-up. In the five years that followed, the 'research' group had significantly lower blood pressure, and 20 per cent fewer deaths, than the GP group.

Most of the extra deaths among the GP care group were from heart attacks and strokes: only about half of them were actually given antihypertensive drugs.

The doctors who conducted both these studies concluded that mild hypertension should be treated as actively as possible. They made several extra points, too. Professor Austin Doyle, of Melbourne University, stressed the importance of treating mild hypertension before it damaged 'end-organs' such as the heart, brain and kidneys. The second point was that most of the patients on placebo in the Australian trial did have satisfactory falls in their blood pressure. He put this down to the better care they were receiving by just being on the trial and being aware that they needed to do something themselves to improve their blood pressure. They had made personal efforts to do so, such as losing excess weight, cutting down on salt, stopping smoking, exercising more and relaxing more.

The big difference in illness and deaths between the two groups of patients came when the diastolic pressure fell below 90 mmHg, however. Such a fall was rare on placebo alone.

Dr Herbert Langford of the University of Mississippi, who reported the US results, stressed that the differences in the rates of death and illness could be explained largely on the finding that those receiving the extra care were known to have stuck more closely to their doctors' instruction and to have taken their drugs more regularly.

Strikingly, among all the 10,000 patients in the two trials, not one death or serious illness was attributable to a side effect of a drug. So not only were the drugs effective, they were also safer than expected. Minor side effects were reported, but no more than on any long-term drug treatment, and very few more than those reported on placebo.

The US researchers had not expected such a large drop in deaths in merely five years. Spread nationwide, such a saving would prevent tens of thousands of deaths each year. The Australians calculated that in their population of (then) 12 million, if all cases of mild hypertension were treated, there would be 7,000 fewer cases of stroke, heart attack and renal failure, and 2,000 fewer deaths each year. These figures would translate to 9,000 fewer deaths in the UK.

There have been hundreds of studies of antihypertensive treatments since 1982, all of them confirming the initial results. Probably the two most important, which finally led to worldwide acceptance of the importance of lowering blood pressure, were published in *The Lancet* on 31 March and 7 April 1990. They reported the work of doctors in the UK, New Zealand and the USA on 42,000 adults with high blood pressure, followed for between six and 25 years.

The first study, on 5,000 patients, showed that reducing the diastolic pressure by only 5 mmHg lowered rates of stroke by 34 per cent and heart attack rate by 21 per cent. The corresponding figures for a 10 mmHg fall were 56 per cent for stroke and 37 per cent for heart attack.

The second report, written by the same group of doctors but this time giving the data for 37,000 patients, showed that the protection against stroke and heart attack became significant within two years of starting treatment, strokes being reduced by 42 per cent and heart attacks by 14 per cent. In the longer term, the stroke risk continued to be cut by around 40 per cent and the fall in heart attack rates stabilized at around 20 to 25 per cent.

Since these reports, which have been confirmed again and again as newer drugs have been put to the test, all doctors routinely screen their patients for early rises in blood pressure, and are meticulous in making sure that whenever hypertension is diagnosed, no matter how mild, it is managed correctly. Even when the blood pressure is only marginally raised, each drop of 2 per cent in average pressure is linked to a 5 per cent drop in risk of a heart attack or stroke.

So how should we go about treating hypertension? The first priority, all the experts agree, is not medication. Everyone with high blood pressure will improve to some extent by changing his or her lifestyle. Some will even improve so much that they will not need drugs. However, it is usually very difficult, as the Australians found, to bring the diastolic pressure below the optimal target of 90 mmHg without drugs. So don't be surprised if your doctor insists on you taking daily antihypertensive drugs even if your blood pressure is not particularly high.

Drugs to control high blood pressure

The next few paragraphs are about drugs that control high blood pressure, but this isn't a catalogue for choosing your own treatment. Of course, today the doctor–patient relationship is a partnership. The old 'doctor knows best' attitude has gone, but decisions on what to prescribe must still be based on good evidence, and your doctor, who works with the British Hypertension Society (BHS) guidelines, has access to that evidence. So be guided by your doctor on what is best for you as an individual with high blood pressure and chronic kidney disease. Of course, have your input on the decision to prescribe, especially if you feel uncomfortable or have side effects with a particular drug or combination of drugs.

Normal blood pressure is maintained by the co-ordination of the different bodily physical and chemical systems explained at the beginning of this chapter. When it is too high that co-ordination has been lost. The different classes of drugs to restore normal blood pressure act on these different systems: your doctor will explain how they do so and why they are used. It is enough here to list them, so that if you need your pressure to be lowered you can recognize the type you have been asked to take. The decision is your doctor's, but it is good to know as much about your particular prescription as possible.

The list (in 2011) comprises:

- diuretics
- beta-blockers
- angiotensin-converting enzyme (ACE) inhibitors
- angiotensin II (ATII) blockers

- calcium-channel blockers
- alpha-1 blockers
- centrally acting agents
- vasodilators
- others best classed as miscellaneous.

If your systolic blood pressure is persistently 140 mmHg or above, and/or your diastolic pressure is 90 mmHg or above, after strenuous efforts to reduce them by other means, you should have drug treatment to lower them. The choice of drug depends on your particular circumstances.

We usually start with a single drug for a week or two, then add another drug in combination treatment if it hasn't brought the pressure down to the target level. If over the next few weeks the combined treatment doesn't control the pressure, the regimen is rethought. Your drugs may be replaced by a new combination, or your initial drug doses may be increased, or a new drug is added.

Do accept that finding you have high blood pressure is hardly ever an emergency. It can take weeks to control. So don't worry if your pressure is not quickly brought into the normal range.

There are a few exceptions to this rule. In a very few people, severe high blood pressure causes symptoms (like dizziness, loss of vision, weakness of one side, severe headaches, chest pains) that indicate they may soon become ill. In their case, emergency admission to hospital is arranged and appropriate measures taken to bring their blood pressure down. Our GP guidelines advise that we start treatment immediately if the systolic pressure is at 220 mmHg or above and/or the diastolic is at or above 120 mmHg. We have more leeway when the initial levels are lower. If you find that you don't feel as well as you should after starting on your antihypertensive drug, report it to your doctor. The 'off-feeling' may be a side effect of your drug, and it can often be managed by dropping the dose for a while or changing to another drug or combination. The current target for everyone is 120/75–80 mmHg, but if you can manage to keep it around the 125/85 mmHg mark, you are doing well.

Keep taking the pills

You may be tempted to stop the treatment because you feel better without the pills. That is understandable if your blood pressure hasn't made you feel ill in the first place and the treatment has side effects. A diuretic, for example, may make you run to the toilet every few hours, and that can be socially inconvenient. Or a beta-blocker may make you wheeze. Or an ACE inhibitor may cause a cough.

But don't succumb to the temptation to stop them without first talking to your doctor. You must learn either to tolerate the side effects or to organize your drugs so that the side effects are minimized or abolished. That can mean something as simple as changing the time of day you take your drugs, or changing their relationship with meals, lowering the dose or changing the drug. Do what you can to ease the side effect without risking a rise in pressure, which is almost inevitable if you stop the tablets.

If you don't take your medicines regularly as advised, your blood pressure will not be under full control. If you don't keep your appointments to have your pressure checked – another common failing – you won't know whether the drugs are working to their best effect. Depend on it that your blood pressure will not tell you that it is rising. You may feel better than you did but have a much higher blood pressure and be heading for a stroke, so don't take the risk. Accept that you have to control your blood pressure for the rest of your life, to help prevent, avoid or delay a heart attack, stroke or dementia.

If you do tend to forget to take your pills despite your best intentions, turn them into a daily routine, like brushing your teeth or setting your bedside alarm. Wear a watch with a 12-hour or once-a-day alarm to remind you of your pill times, wherever you are and whatever you are doing.

The introduction in the last few years of easy-to-use blood pressure measuring machines (sphygmomanometers) has helped many people to follow their pressure at home. They find that readings taken a few times a week keep them confident that their treatment is working, or can detect early a rise that needs to be discussed with their medical team. I must say here that I have found that some of the new 'sphygmos' give erratic readings that don't correlate with our standard machines in the surgery. So if you are thinking of buying one, please check its accuracy with your doctor's or nurse's sphygmo, to make sure it is accurate. You should choose one that employs a cuff around the upper arm.

To summarize

This chapter has been about high blood pressure and why it is important, if you wish to lower your risk of eventual dementia, to keep it under control. The aim is to protect the delicate tissues of your arteries, throughout your body and particularly in your brain, from the effects of higher than normal pressure.

However, your arteries also need protection from another coronary- and stroke-producing menace, cholesterol. A high cholesterol level is the building block for atheroma, mentioned earlier in this chapter. If yours is high, you will almost certainly have been advised to lower it. The next chapter explains why cholesterol is so important.

9

Dementia provokers 4 – your cholesterol risk

To understand the role of blood lipids like cholesterol in protecting our circulation and our kidneys, we need to know more about the 'good' and 'bad' lipids, how they come to be in the blood at all, and what they do.

Why do we need cholesterol, considering that it does so much damage, as in atheroma, to our arteries? I can best answer that by posing a 'Trivial Pursuit'- type question. What is the fattest organ in the body – the one that contains the highest proportion of fat in comparison with the two other essential foodstuffs, protein or glucose? The answer is the brain.

The brain needs a lot of fat, because fat is an essential component of nerve cells and their 'insulating' covering, a substance called myelin. Without myelin separating nerve cell fibres from each other, the electrical signal that runs along the fibres would dissipate into the surrounding tissues and the nervous system would not work. This is, in fact, the problem in people with multiple sclerosis: their myelin sheaths deteriorate, and their nerves fail to work.

So we need to transport fats around our bodies to keep our organs healthy and working to maximum capacity. We do that by using the 'family' of fats, one group of which is cholesterol-based.

Cholesterol has a complex chemical structure, the details of which are outside the remit of this book. Its 'building blocks' are derived from fatty acids that we obtain in the first place from fats in our food. The story goes like this. We swallow food containing fat or oil. These are digested into fatty acids and pass to the liver, which turns them into cholesterol. This passes into the bloodstream, where it is transported into the tissues that need it, and is converted into the type of fat needed by the organ. For example, it can be myelin for nervous tissue, 'phospholipids' (fats attached to phosphate molecules) or 'lipoproteins' (fats combined with proteins) for specialist jobs in brain and nerve cells or for breast milk, or simpler fats for storage around our gut or under the skin.

Fats and why we need them

Fat storage is a relic from our hundreds of thousands of years as hunter–gatherers, when we had to face many times of near-famine. We ate as much as we could in times of plenty so that we could live on our fat stores in times of near-starvation. Our usual immediate source of energy is glucose, which we make in our gut from the digestion of sugars and starches, but we have very limited capacity to store it. In fact, glucose is stored as a substance called glycogen in some muscles and the liver, but all our body's supply of glycogen can quickly be used up when we exert ourselves. From then on we have to use stored fats as our energy source.

We inherited from our Stone Age ancestors a very efficient system for storing fats, so that they can be used as fuel for our muscles, brain and other organs when we have nothing to eat or have used up our glucose and glycogen. Conditions ten thousand or more years ago probably kept our ancestors thin, meaning that they used up all the fat they could consume in their daily lives. Today, everyone in the Global North has enough to eat. If we do not use up in energetic activity all the fat and glucose we eat each day, then we have to store it, and almost all of it is stored as fat. Even with normal body shapes, with no obesity, the average woman is 18 per cent and the average man 10 per cent fat.

However, fewer and fewer of us have normal body shapes. We exercise far less than we used to, and we eat and drink more. Today, by the time we reach 50 years old, nearly half of us, men and women, are overweight enough to be described as 'obese'. That means someone is at least 30 per cent fat, and perhaps a lot more.

Where does that fat go, and what does it consist of? We may put it on our waists, our hips or our backs (in a 'buffalo hump'), or space it fairly equally under the skin all round our torso and limbs. It is also laid down in the walls of our arteries, as streaks and plaques. Classically, people are described as 'apples' (with fat mainly around the waist and inside the abdomen) or 'pears' (with most of the fat around the hips and bottom). There is some evidence that the apples are more prone to heart attacks than pears, because they lay more fat in their artery walls than the pears do, but any form of obesity raises the risks.

'Good' and 'bad' cholesterol

However, the message of this chapter isn't just about obesity. There are some (not many) obese people with relatively low 'bad' cholesterol levels in their blood, and there are thin people (again, not many) who have high 'bad' cholesterol levels. And of the two, those with the high cholesterol levels, whether they are fat or thin, are more likely to have a heart attack or stroke and, consequently, vascular dementia.

Which is where we must explain about 'bad' and 'good' cholesterol. The medical name for fat of any sort is 'lipid'. 'Blood lipid level' is the term for the amount of fats in your venous blood, taken usually from a vein in your arm. The lipids we are most concerned about fall into two main categories, cholesterol and triglyceride. However, they don't float about in the blood on their own. Most molecules of cholesterol and triglyceride in the blood are transported around attached to proteins, so they are called 'lipoprotein complexes'. We identify the different types of lipoprotein complex by spinning the plasma (blood from which the red cells have been removed) in a centrifuge. That separates out the different lipoproteins from each other according to how dense (heavy) they are.

There are:

- very low density lipoproteins (VLDLs)
- low density lipoproteins (LDLs)
- high density lipoproteins (HDLs).

Triglyceride (TG) is usually carried in VLDLs, and cholesterol in LDLs or HDLs. In your blood test report, TC means total cholesterol, LDL-C means the LDL-cholesterol level, and the same goes for VLDL-C and HDL-C. TG stands for triglyceride level. Don't confuse TC with TG.

The body attaches fats to proteins (to form lipoproteins) because this is the only way in which lipids can be transported across the healthy small artery walls. Combined with protein, the fat molecule is soluble and is easy for the artery walls to handle. As a free fat in the blood, either as cholesterol or triglyceride, it remains relatively insoluble, cannot cross the intact endothelium (the internal arterial wall lining) and remains in the blood. However, if the endothelium is damaged it is a different story. Without an intact layer of healthy artery lining cells to protect the blood-vessel wall, the fats and triglyceride can pass into the wall, where they are laid down as solid deposits, helping to form the structure of plaques.

Your blood test result will indicate your levels of triglyceride, HDL and LDL, along with your total cholesterol. Local hospital laboratories all over the world measure blood lipid levels in their own populations, and relate the results in each individual to their normal range. The normal range differs from country to country, within areas in the same country, and even within populations in different districts in the same city. So it is difficult to be precise in a book like this on what is 'normal' and what is 'high' for you.

However, specialists in diseases of blood vessels and lipid disorders have defined what they see as acceptable generally for everyone. Everyone with a blood lipid 'profile' that causes concern is given a general diagnosis of dyslipidaemia. The term simply means abnormal levels of fat in the blood. If you have a higher than normal level of TC or LDL-C this is called hypercholesterolaemia (from *hyper*, 'too much', cholesterol, and *aemia*, meaning 'in the blood'). Too high a TG level is called hypertriglyceridaemia, and when both cholesterol and TG are raised, it is called combined hyperlipidaemia.

Some people have low HDL-C levels but their other lipids are in the normal range: they are diagnosed as having dyslipidaemia. However, a low HDL-C almost always goes with hypertriglyceridaemia, so low HDL-C on its own is relatively rare. All these types of dyslipidaemia may be inborn (inherited with your genes) or 'secondary' (brought on by lifestyle), or a combination of both.

Crucial to the recognition of dyslipidaemias is that they are very strongly related to your risk of having heart attacks and strokes.

In particular, the worse your hypercholesterolaemia or hypertrigly-ceridaemia, or both, the higher is your risk of succumbing to one of these catastrophes. The risk rises throughout the range of blood cholesterol, from the lowest of all to the highest, and the slope is a steep one.

We measure lipid levels in the UK in millimoles of each type of lipid per litre (mmol/l) of blood. A man with a total plasma cholesterol (TC) level of 5.2 mmol/l has half the risk of coronary heart disease (angina and heart attack) of one with a TC of 6.5 mmol/l and only a quarter of the risk of a man with a TC of 7.8 mmol/l. Put another way, if you reduce your TC from 7.8 to 5.2 you will reduce your heart attack risk by three-quarters.

This is not guesswork. It has been proved time and time again in populations within countries and in comparisons between countries. Countries with low TC levels like Japan (average around 4.9 mmol/l) have about 60 coronary and stroke deaths per 100,000 people per year; in those with averages above 6 mmol/l, like my own country, Scotland, the corresponding figure is 600. Finland used to have similar figures – ten times those of Japan – but since its government initiated a huge healthy lifestyle campaign both the TC levels and the numbers of deaths have plummeted. The relationship between TC levels and deaths from heart attacks is constant for almost every country. Take Poland, with a TC average 5.5 and a 'heart' death rate of 280, or Germany with 5.7 and 320, and England with 6.5 and 470. One 'outlier', or exception, is France, with an average TC of 5.8 and a death rate of only 135. That is almost certainly explained by the regular consumption in France of red wine, which seems to protect against deposition of fats in artery walls.

However, a rise in TC alone does not explain all the cholesterol-related deaths. When concerns were raised in the 1950s about the steep increase in heart disease, health experts all over the world started to study their own populations 'prospectively'. That is, they selected healthy people for close follow-up over many years, having first measured their blood lipid profiles. Some were left to follow their usual lifestyles without interference, while other trials promoted what was thought then to be a healthier lifestyle for hearts to some subjects and not to others. The goal was to follow as many as possible to their eventual deaths, and to record their age at death and the cause.

The results of most of these studies were published in the 1980s, and they became the basis for almost all we do about managing high blood lipid levels today. Certainly they provided the motivation to doctors to ensure that their patients should keep their lipid profiles as healthy as possible.

All the studies confirmed that men with higher TC levels were more likely to die from heart attacks and strokes than those with lower TC levels. But in each study there were substantial numbers of men with low TC levels who still died early. This was true in countries in continental Europe, the USA and the UK. In the British Regional Heart Study (conducted by A.G. Shaper and colleagues and reported in *Journal of Epidemiology and Community Health*, 1985, volume 39, pages 197–209), one in five of the men recorded as having serious or fatal heart attacks or strokes had TCs below 6 mmol/l. They were in the lowest 40 per cent of the range of TC results.

Why did so many people with relatively low TCs die? There are several ways of explaining this. Perhaps a TC of 6 mmol/l is still far too high for safety. It is certainly very much higher than the average Japanese TC. We should probably aim for a TC under 5 mmol/l. Or there may be other aspects of their lipids, such as a high TG and LDL-C, with a low HDL-C, that were not measured in the studies. Or other factors, such as high blood pressure, smoking habit and diabetes, may have played their part.

In fact, all these explanations are true. Why should some lipids, like LDL-C and TG, be thought to be 'bad' for us, and HDL-C be thought to be 'good'? Let's go back to the idea of fats being deposited into the blood-vessel walls, where they cause plaques of atheroma, and eventually block or rupture the artery. How does that happen? The most recent view is as follows.

The liver receives fatty acids, as described on page 82, from the bowel after our digestion forms them by breaking down fats in our food. The liver cells then start the process of turning the fatty acids into triglyceride and cholesterol. The combination of the two with protein forms VLDL-C. This is the most suitable form of fat for release from the liver into the bloodstream. Once there, it is then ready for delivery to the smallest blood vessels for transport across the small artery walls into the tissues. On the way, the VLDL-C is progressively enriched with more cholesterol, which makes the molecules more dense, forming LDL-C. The endothelium is therefore faced with VLDL-C and LDL-C, which it must carry across into the tissues beyond, so that the fat can be used for the building and energy processes described earlier.

So far, so good. But what happens if there is too much VLDL-C and LDL-C? Some of it circulates back to the liver, where it is taken up by the liver cells and stored for future use. Some of it is taken up by fat storage cells. But a sizeable proportion of it remains in the connective tissue layer just beyond the artery lining cells, where it is treated by the body as an irritant and 'scavenged' by white blood cells called to the site to deal with it. The white cells fill with cholesterol and become 'foam' cells, so named because under the microscope they look as if they are filled with foam.

Foam cells do not survive long. They die, releasing free cholesterol into the artery wall. If this state continues, platelets (tiny solid cell remnants that circulate in the blood) are attracted to the area, and form tiny 'thromboses' on the surface. This is the beginning of a plaque. High VLDL-C (containing mainly triglyceride) and high LDL-C (containing mainly cholesterol) levels are therefore a recipe for forming and maintaining and enlarging plaques. They are justifiably called 'bad' lipids.

Where does HDL-C fit into this? The endothelium does try to heal itself and to get rid of the cholesterol and triglyceride gathering like a microscopic blackhead around it. The only way it can do that is to make the LDL-C and the VLDL-C even denser. Only by collecting the fats into high-density lipoprotein masses, by turning VLDL-C and LDL-C into HDL-C, can the arteries manage to extrude the fats from the deposits in their walls back into the bloodstream. Once in the bloodstream, the only organ to take it up in any serious amount is the liver, which can then turn it into bile and excrete it.

So HDL-C is the body's answer to excessive fat deposits: it is made by the endothelium to protect itself. A high HDL-C means that there is a good turnover of lipids in the body, in the direction of lowering fatty deposits in the artery walls. HDL-C is justifiably the 'good' cholesterol.

So what does all this mean?

How can we bring all these facts about cholesterol and blood lipids together? The first message is that the higher your total cholesterol, the more likely you are to have a heart attack and/or stroke, and to have it earlier rather than later in your life. The second message is that TC is not the only risk. TC is only a rough guide. Within it are VLDL-C (mainly triglyceride), LDL-C (mainly cholesterol) and HDL-C. Raise the first two and lower the third, and you make a heart attack and/or stroke more likely. Lower the first two and raise the third, and you reduce your chance of a heart attack and/or stroke.

Most of today's management of people with high cholesterol is now devoted to lowering TG and LDL-C and if possible raising HDL-C at the same time. How we do that is described in Chapter 11.

To summarize cholesterol and your arteries

The higher your blood cholesterol level, the more fat is likely to be deposited in the walls of your arteries, as plaques. The longer it continues to be high, the greater the number of plaques and the bigger they will be. The more plaques in your arteries, the higher your chance of having a heart attack and/or stroke. It is as simple as that. Lower your cholesterol level, and you will substantially lower that chance.

Obviously you mustn't depend on lowering cholesterol alone. You must also tackle other aspects of your life that harm your arteries. If you have high blood pressure that is not well controlled, then those muscles wrapped round your arteries will grow thicker and narrow your arteries, making a blockage much more likely. It will also put extra strain on areas of plaque, so that they can split asunder, tear the artery wall and cause a bleed. In the brain that is a 'haemorrhagic' stroke.

I have already written about smoking, but it still makes sense to add a little about it here. If you smoke, then you directly damage your arterial walls with each inhalation you take. The thousand or so damaging chemicals in smoke pass into your blood, and they poison the very delicate single layer of cells, the endothelium, that lines every artery. Smokers have far fewer functioning active artery lining cells than non-smokers. This leads to many problems for the circulation. For a start, they cannot give the signal to the muscle layer to relax, so that the calibre of the tube through which the blood has to flow is greatly reduced. That means less oxygen getting through to the tissues beyond. In fact, smoking already compromises the oxygen supply to the artery wall because so many smokers' red cells carry carbon monoxide, rather than oxygen, around the body. And you can't use carbon monoxide for energy! It is the same deadly poison that used to kill people when they put their heads in gas ovens using the old town gas.

Smoking also harms the arteries by promoting blood clotting. It increases the blood levels of a substance, fibrinogen, that is the most powerful natural blood-clotting agent. It also makes the blood stickier so that elements of it called platelets stick to the artery walls and to each other far more easily. Once stuck together they stay stuck. Clots develop on top of heaps of stuck-together platelets.

Then there is nicotine itself. Smokers of even one cigarette a day put enough nicotine in their blood to cause the muscles around the arteries to contract – making the arteries, already under an onslaught, even narrower. If you were deliberately to try to design a drug that would kill people with a heart attack or stroke, you could not possibly do better than tobacco.

Finally, if you have diabetes, constantly higher than normal levels of glucose in your blood, along with high blood pressure, can also damage the arteries. So do follow your strict plan of diabetes and blood pressure control.

The message of this chapter, therefore, is to look on your arteries in the same way as you look on your brain, lungs, heart, liver and kidneys. Most of us dread the thought of our brain going in old age, and ending up with dementia. So we try to stave it off by keeping it active. We know about our lungs, and how smoking affects them. We all know of the messages about a healthy heart – no one could have missed the promotion of healthy eating, such as five portions of fruit and vegetables a day, with oily fish and perhaps red wine thrown in. Every so often a celebrity is shown to have liver disease bad enough to need a transplant because of his or her excessive drinking (footballer George Best springs to mind). But how many of us know that we need to look after our arteries? Or how important cholesterol and other fats in our blood are to keeping them healthy? Yet keeping our arteries healthy is the key to keeping all the other organs healthy, too.

10

Lowering cholesterol

If you have a raised cholesterol level you are probably taking a lipid-lowering drug, and you perhaps wonder whether it is doing more harm than good. This is a common problem for people who have few, if any, symptoms of disease, yet who are told they must take drugs for the rest of their life if they are to avoid future illness. They naturally fear that taking a drug for years may have an unexpected damaging side effect. Would it be worth stopping the drug and taking the chance that they won't get the predicted heart attack or stroke?

So this chapter first sets out the recommendations by the European Joint Task Force (a group of distinguished specialists in lipid disorders) on who should have lipid-lowering drugs. It then gives the evidence from trials that caused the task force to come to the decisions it did, and leaves you to decide on whether the benefits of the drugs outweigh the potential drawbacks.

Who shouldn't and who should be offered drug treatment

Unless you already have been ill with, or are showing early symptoms of heart disease, you do not need drugs if you have mild or moderate hypercholesterolaemia (raised cholesterol level) that has started to reverse after you have changed your lifestyle.

According to the European Joint Task Force, you do need drug treatment if you:

- are a high-risk patient, i.e. someone who already has shown signs of heart or kidney disease;
- have other risk factors such as high blood pressure;

- are at high risk through special risk factors, such as having high lipoprotein(a) or high fibrinogen levels in your blood (both indicate fairly severe risk to your arteries);
- have hypercholesterolaemia that has not responded to changes in lifestyle designed to lower your cholesterol;
- have inherited ('familial') hyperlipidaemia, with relatives who died early, as it is unlikely to respond to lifestyle changes and carries a high risk of heart attack and stroke;
- have any severe form of dyslipidaemia, or evidence of coronary disease along with mild or moderate dyslipidaemia.

You will gather from these guidelines that almost everyone with a high cholesterol or evidence of artery disease is eligible for drug treatment. The Task Force was convinced by the results of trials of the drugs that they provide much more benefit than they do harm. Here is some of the evidence on which that judgement was based.

The evidence for drugs

The Air Force/Texas Coronary Atherosclerosis Prevention Study (AFCAPS/TexCAPS)

This study was reported to the American Heart Association in 1997. It followed 6,605 men and women with mildly raised cholesterol levels, but no initial evidence of heart disease, given either a 'statin' (lovastatin) or placebo.

The study was stopped early because of the far greater 'event rate' (numbers of people with heart attacks and strokes) among those taking the placebo than in those on the statin. On the statin there were 40 per cent fewer fatal and non-fatal heart attacks, 32 per cent fewer serious attacks of angina and a 33 per cent reduction in the numbers of people needing emergency coronary artery surgery. Women, older people, smokers, people with high blood pressure and those with diabetes all benefited from the statin, and the improvement was seen even in those with the mildest rise in blood lipid levels.

Atorvastatin Versus Revascularization Treatments (AVERT)

The 341 people who entered AVERT all had known coronary artery disease with angina. They all had angiograms that showed they had narrowing of at least one coronary artery. Then they were allocated randomly to either medical treatment with atorvastatin or to angioplasty (in which a balloon-tipped catheter is used to expand the narrowed coronary segment). Angioplasty is regarded as the standard treatment of coronary artery narrowing in people with angina. It is usually highly successful and has been a great addition to our ability to treat people with angina. It is routinely used during heart attacks in specialist hospitals to prevent heart muscle damage.

Of course, angioplasties do not guarantee prevention of further attacks of angina or even full heart attacks (in which an artery is completely blocked and the area of heart muscle beyond the blockage dies). Atorvastatin turned out to be more effective than angioplasty. There were 36 per cent fewer new 'cardiac' episodes (attacks of angina or heart attacks) and the time from start of treatment to the next event was longer on the atorvastatin treatment than after the angioplasties. TC, LDL-C and TG levels were all lower on atorvastatin than after angioplasty, and there were fewer serious side effects of treatment on atorvastatin than after angioplasty.

The authors concluded that atorvastatin may help doctors to postpone or even completely avoid angioplasty procedures in some patients with mild or moderate coronary artery disease.

Cholesterol and Recurrent Events (CARE) Study

CARE followed people with high LDL-C levels who also had already had heart attacks. It enrolled 4,159 patients with TC below 6.2 mmol/l and LDL-C of 3 to 4.5 mmol/l. They would have been borderline candidates for drugs if they had not had a heart attack. Half were given pravastatin and half placebo, and they were followed for five years. There were 24 per cent fewer heart attacks on pravastatin than on placebo. There was also 26 per cent less need for coronary artery bypass surgery, a 23 per cent reduction in angioplasty and a 31 per cent reduction in stroke.

Interestingly, CARE showed that women responded to pravastatin better than men, with a bigger drop in heart attacks, strokes and the need for surgery, particularly in those with higher initial LDL-C values.

Long-term Intervention with Pravastatin in Ischaemic Disease (LIPID)

Doctors in 87 centres in Australia and New Zealand in the 1990s gave more than 9,000 patients either pravastatin or placebo. They all had coronary artery disease and had been previously admitted to hospital because of a heart attack or an attack of severe angina. LIPID had to be stopped early, after six years, because of the obvious advantage enjoyed by the statin-treated group. Those given pravastatin showed reductions of 18 per cent in TC, 25 per cent in LDL-C and 12 per cent in TG. There was an increase of 6 per cent in HDL-C. Linked with these changes were reductions of 24 per cent in deaths due to heart events and an overall reduction in deaths from all causes of 22 per cent. People concerned with the costs of prescribing statins to so many patients were reassured by the news that the statin group needed 20 per cent fewer angioplasties and bypass operations. This made the overall costs of drug treatment less than the costs of no drugs coupled with the need for patient 'rescue' with extra heart surgery.

The Scandinavian Simvastatin Survival Study (4S)

This was one of the earlier studies of the use of statins in people with hypercholesterolaemia. It concentrated on patients with total cholesterol levels between 5.5 and 8.0 mmol/l, and for five years followed 4,444 patients allocated to simvastatin or placebo. By the end of the trial there were 34 per cent fewer major heart problems on simvastatin than on placebo. This study showed that for each fall of 1 per cent in TC, the risk of a major cardiac event (MCE) fell by 1.9 per cent, and a 1 per cent fall in LDL-C led to a reduction of 1.7 per cent in MCEs.

West of Scotland Coronary Prevention Study (WOSCOPS)

I must admit bias towards this study because it was conducted in my home area, and I know some of the GPs and the men who took part in it.

WOSCOPS followed 6,595 men who had never had a heart attack, giving them either pravastatin or placebo. Pravastatin certainly worked: there were 36 per cent fewer severe heart events on it than on placebo. However, the fall could not be related to changes in cholesterol levels from their starting point or to the cholesterol levels on treatment. The authors felt that the benefits of pravastatin were not due to reduction in LDL-C alone. They did show that the men with higher than average TG levels (more than 1.6 mmol/l) benefited more from the statin than men with higher than average total cholesterol levels (more than 7 mmol/l), although both groups gained substantial benefit.

Other studies

The Stockholm Ischaemic Heart Disease Secondary Prevention Study supported this conclusion that lowering TG levels offered considerable benefits. In its patients whose TG was lowered by more than 30 per cent, the deaths from heart disease fell by a massive 60 per cent.

This chapter could go on and on relating the different trials of drugs in hyperlipidaemia, but enough is enough. On the use of lipid-lowering agents in people with hyperlipidaemias of all types, the defence rests. All the trials showed benefit outweighing the risk of adverse events. The current lipid-lowering drugs are described in the next chapter.

11

Drugs to lower cholesterol

Drugs that improve blood lipid levels have been a huge success. The trials listed in the previous chapter are only some among many that have shown that they do what they claim to – they lower cholesterol and triglyceride levels, and in doing so they prevent deaths from heart attacks and strokes in the people most vulnerable to them.

However, the best known of these drugs are the statins, and they may not be the correct drugs for everyone with a lipid problem. Today there are four 'lipid-lowering' types of drug – the statins, fibrates, bile-acid sequestrants and nicotinic acid.

Statins – or HMG-CoA reductase inhibitors

The statins in current use include atorvastatin, fluvastatin, pravastatin and simvastatin. They hit the headlines in 2001 when cerivastatin was withdrawn after reports of unacceptably high numbers of cases of muscle pains, especially when given with fibrates.

Statins work by blocking an enzyme, HMG-CoA reductase, which is involved in the making of cholesterol in the liver. They are most effective, therefore, in reducing LDL-C, but are less effective in lowering high TG levels. Nevertheless, they do reduce TG by between 15 and 40 per cent, depending on the dose. Doses range up to 80 mg per day for atorvastatin, fluvastatin and simvastatin, and up to 40 mg per day for pravastatin.

Most people tolerate statins well. The main problem is with muscles: a few people given statins develop pains in the muscles, often in the shoulder and upper back. If this happens to you, you should stop the drug and report the effect to your doctor. The muscle problem may be made worse (even to the extent that some of the muscle tissues are destroyed in a process called rhabdomyolysis) if the drug is given with fibrates, which are mainly used to lower TG levels. They may also be worsened if you are taking drugs for other illnesses, such as ciclosporin (to prevent transplant rejection), the antibiotic erythromycin and the antifungal ketoconazole.

You will not be prescribed statins if you have liver disease or are a heavy drinker, as they can be toxic to a liver that is showing chronic disease, such as active hepatitis or alcoholic degeneration. Your doctor will take blood for liver function tests before you start on a statin, and repeat the tests every six months.

Other less often reported side effects include headache, abdominal pain, flatulence, diarrhoea, nausea and vomiting. There have been very rare reports of rashes and allergic reactions to statins. Statins combine well with bile-acid sequestrants, but must be used with great care with fibrates or nicotinic acid.

By blocking the HMG-CoA reductase enzyme, statins reduce both LDL-C and VLDL, so that they reduce blood total cholesterol and TG levels while slightly increasing HDL-C. Which one your doctor chooses to use depends a lot on his or her personal experience with this class of drugs. They are probably all similar in effect and side effects. The ones that remain are unlikely to go the way of cerivastatin.

Fibrates

Fibrates include bezafibrate, ciprofibrate, fenofibrate and gemfibrozil. They lower VLDL by blocking its synthesis in the liver, so that they are useful in treating combined hypercholesterolaemia and hypertriglyceridaemia. They may also stimulate the clearance of excess LDL-C from the plasma. All fibrates tend to raise HDL-C, but only by a small amount.

As with the statins, most people have no trouble taking the fibrates. However, there are some reports of nausea, diarrhoea, gallstones, alopecia and muscle weakness with fibrates, and your doctor will wish to monitor the liver regularly. There are rare cases of liver upsets on fibrates. Very great care must be taken if you are considering taking a fibrate with a statin, as the combination can lead to muscle problems. However, there are few problems in prescribing fibrates along with nicotinic acid or bile-acid sequestrants.

Bile-acid sequestrants

There are two current bile-acid sequestrants, cholestyramine and colestipol. They work by binding to the bile acids in the gut, so that these can no longer deliver fats to the liver for processing into new cholesterol and triglyceride. The liver therefore needs to 'suck' cholesterol back into itself from the circulation. This sets up a flow of fats from their deposits in the endothelium through the circulation into the liver. Plasma cholesterol levels therefore fall. However, there may be a downside – VLDL-C and TG levels may rise.

Cholestyramine and colestipol are used in people with raised LDL-C, but not in hypertriglyceridaemia or in people with constipation. Constipation is the main side effect of bile-acid sequestrants, and may be too inconvenient for people to continue with them, although 'bulking' laxatives like Fybogel usually relieves it. Bile-acid sequestrants may reduce the absorption of other important drugs, making them less effective. You should therefore not take them within three hours of taking doses of warfarin (to stop blood clotting), thyroxine (thyroid hormone), diuretics and beta-blockers (usually given for high blood pressure, but sometimes for an abnormal heart rhythm). They may also affect the uptake from the gut of folic acid (given before and during pregnancy, mainly to prevent spina bifida and other spine and brain abnormalities in developing infants) and vitamins A and D.

People taking bile-acid sequestrants should have their blood monitored for possible malabsorption problems (such as anaemia) each year. These drugs can be given with each of the other lipid-lowering drug types.

Nicotinic acid

Nicotinic acid is a vitamin, but the dose used to lower blood lipid levels is much higher than the usual daily need for it. Nicotinic acid reduces the formation of VLDL in the liver, at the same time reducing the level of free fatty acids (the 'building blocks' of cholesterol) in the circulation.

Nicotinic acid decreases VLDL-C and LDL-C, while increasing

HDL-C by a very substantial 15 to 25 per cent. It starts at doses of around 100 to 250 mg, rising gradually to as much as 4.5 to 6 grams daily. Higher doses may cause liver problems.

Its main problem is flushing, which can be reduced by taking an aspirin about 15 to 30 minutes beforehand. Nicotinic acid can add to the effect of blood pressure-lowering drugs, so you should be warned about that if you are asked to take the combination. It can cause gout, a skin condition called acanthosis nigricans and swelling of the retina in the back of the eye, but happily these side effects all disappear when the drug is stopped. People with active liver disease, diabetes (nicotinic acid can raise blood glucose levels) and gout should probably not take nicotinic acid. If you are taking it you should have a blood test to check your liver and blood glucose every six months or so.

It can be given safely with fibrates and bile-acid sequestrants, but not with statins, as it may increase the risk of severe muscle reactions.

Summarizing cholesterol-lowering drugs

By now you will have realized that the choice of cholesterol-lowering drugs, like that for high blood pressure, is wide and can be tailored to your particular needs. So your doctors will choose for you a statin, a fibrate, a bile-acid sequestrant or nicotinic acid. The choice depends on your particular pattern of lipids, as well as your total cholesterol level, and also on how well you tolerate the drug you are given. All have their drawbacks, as well as their benefits, so be prepared to have to change them if they are not right for you.

However, drugs alone aren't the answer. To give yourself the best chance of surviving with your brain as intact as possible, and of avoiding the heart attack to which your high cholesterol makes you vulnerable, you have to live the correct lifestyle, too. The next chapter helps you to do this.

12

And finally – living well

By now, having read about the efforts researchers have made to identify ways in which you might avoid or delay dementia, and the chapters on the dementia provokers, you may need a practical overview on the lifestyle that best suits your needs.

How you live matters a lot. You have already read about smoking and alcohol as dementia provokers. What about exercise and eating? Here we have a more cheerful message.

Exercise

Keeping physically active is an essential. Being a genius intellectually and using your brain while being a couch potato will not protect you against the onset or the fast deterioration of either Alzheimer's or vascular dementia. But being physically energetic may well do so. So if you enjoy intellectual things, don't forget the physical as well. Try to be as fit as you can comfortably be, without going overboard about it.

You think you are fit enough already? Then try the Harvard Step Test. You can do it at home. All you need is a flight of stairs and a watch. Step from the floor on to the second step (miss the first) of the stairs and down again. Try to do this 30 times a minute for four minutes. Time yourself with the watch. You must straighten your knee fully at each step up.

If you get too exhausted to carry on, note down the time that you stopped: it will make a difference to your eventual score. If you have any problems, such as tightness in the chest, stop immediately, rest and tell your doctor about it.

As soon as you finish sit down quietly and take your pulse for a full 30 seconds, starting exactly one minute after you stopped exercising. Write down the number of beats immediately, then repeat the 30-second pulse count and recording twice more, starting two minutes after you stopped the exercise, then a minute later. You can then calculate your recovery index. This is the duration of the exercise in seconds multiplied by 100, divided by double the sum of the three pulse counts.

Take these two examples. Mr A stopped the exercise after 3 minutes 40 seconds (220 seconds) and his respective 30-second pulse rates were 76, 64 and 60. This gives a score of 22,000 divided by 400, or 55. Miss B completed the four minutes and her pulse readings were 66, 57 and 53. She had a score of 68 (24,000 divided by 352).

Mr A was decidedly unfit. Miss B was fairly fit, but could do better. Try the exercise yourself. If your score is 60 or less you need to be much fitter. You are only 'fair' between 61 and 70, 'good' between 71 and 80, and 'very fit' between 81 and 90. If you score over 90 you are probably already an athlete in training.

Improving your fitness would help your cardiovascular system, and by association help prevent cardiovascular disease, including dementia. But you don't have to jog or run to do it. Just walk more, to begin with. If you are a commuter, walk to the station whenever the weather is reasonable, or walk for a bus stop or two before getting on. Take stairs rather than a lift or escalator. Go by foot to any place within a mile or so, rather than by car. Do, rather than watch, things in your spare time. Go swimming, cycling or walking at weekends. Try gardening or DIY. Any activity is better than none.

Above all, do enough exercise to make yourself reasonably out of breath three times a week or more. If you think you might enjoy running, try it, but wear the right footwear if you intend to use pavements. If an exercise bores you, try something else.

Don't take it too seriously, either. Few people are worse than exercise bores who constantly talk about their times or speeds. Don't buy a stopwatch – competition shouldn't figure high in your leisure time. The idea is to get away from stress, not add to it. A four-mile walk will get you as fit as if you run the distance in half the time.

Exercise won't kill you. As long as you are sensible about starting, you don't need to consult your doctor beforehand. There are even exercises for people in heart failure, and they feel much the better for them.

Choose your exercise wisely. Don't opt for exercises such as weightlifting: the action of lifting weights or straining muscles while holding your breath is harmful, not beneficial. 'Explosive' sports like squash may also not be right for you. Golf and tennis are more leisurely and probably more acceptable, but if you are new to them take lessons first. Few 'rabbits' last long unless they make rapid progress in their skills.

Daily exercise is all very well, but rest is important, too. You must have your rest periods to let the muscles recover fully. So save two days a week for resting. If you are ill, don't try to keep up with your exercise schedule, particularly if you have a virus infection such as flu or a cold. Never exercise until you are exhausted. Keep it moderate so that you continue to enjoy it. Mixing your activities, too, will help you enjoy the new life more. Take your pick of golf, tennis, cycling, swimming, jogging or simply walking the dog. Do several of them. The variety will give extra interest.

Will the exercise actually improve your chances of avoiding multi-infarct dementia? All the studies of people who exercise suggest that it should. People who exercise regularly are less likely to smoke and overeat, tend not to have high blood pressure and have lower blood cholesterol levels than the rest of the population. Their risk of a heart attack is much less than that of couch potatoes.

Exercise also postpones the onset of old age, and when you do get there you will have a straighter back, better neck movements, more mobile joints and more muscle bulk. Older people who are fitter physically feel less depressed and isolated from others. Women who exercise (and men, too) are much less likely to suffer fractures from osteoporosis – a high-risk complication for women.

Once you start your new life of physical activity, how will you know if you are getting fitter? You will feel better in yourself, and be more alert and happier. If you want to prove the benefit beyond doubt, try the Harvard Step Test again after a week of the new you. Your score will have risen dramatically. It will be easier to continue for the full four minutes, and your pulse rates will be much slower. Aim for the mid-70 region, and keep around that mark. You don't have to be an Olympic athlete to be fit and well.

Eating well

All you need to help yourself avoid dementia is a well-balanced and varied eating habit (I hesitate to call it a diet, as that suggests you are restricted in eating by your illness, and that's the wrong view to take). So eat a variety of foods, but try to make them as fresh as possible. Many processed foods contain far too much salt and, as we learned a few chapters ago, that tends to increase your body's fluid volume and blood pressure, both of which are damaging to your kidneys.

Be wary of salt

Here I must introduce Dr Mark MacGregor, Director of our Renal Unit at Crosshouse Hospital in Ayrshire. He was especially helpful to me in preparing my book *Living with Kidney Disease* (Sheldon Press, 2008). However, his advice on eating is just as applicable to people without any evidence of kidney disease, so I reproduce it here.

He told me that the UK government's recommendation for salt intake is less than 5 grams (100 millimoles) a day. This is too high for his kidney patients, but it is also probably difficult for the rest of us to be able to buy foods that will allow us to eat so little salt in a day. We should eat fresh produce rather than processed foods, but it isn't always easy to do so. Salt is everywhere, says Dr MacGregor – in milk, bread and confectionery.

Happily, most supermarket chains now produce a healthy eating guide and label foods with their salt content. The Co-op and Marks and Spencer led the way and I unashamedly recommend them to you. I must admit here to a certain attachment to the Co-op, as my earliest memories include going for the 'messages' (the Scots term for shopping) for my grandmother. I share with Baroness Betty Boothroyd the memory of the family 'divi' number – she apparently did the same for her grandparents.

Sadly for you, take-aways, whether they come from the pizza parlour, the 'Indian' or the chippy, are full of salt, so, apart from the occasional treat, it's best to cook your own, using ingredients that you know won't push up your salt levels, and with them your total body fluid volume and blood pressure. As for the big fast-food joints – KFC, Burger King, McDonald's and the like – don't bother.

Enjoy!

Most of all, enjoy your choice of food. Have plenty of fresh vegetables and fruit, meat, fish, cereals and dairy products, prepared in a delicious way so that you enjoy them. There isn't a secret ingredient that will enhance your chance of avoiding dementia, nor is there one that will worsen your risk. The only advice on eating I can really give is not to eat too much! Obesity is a no-no, as it links with those high cholesterol and high blood pressure levels. Moderate your drinking with your meals, so that you can enjoy the complementary tastes together. And eat regularly with friends in a convivial atmosphere.

Most of all, now that you are on the right path to avoiding dementia, you can forget all about it, and enjoy the rest of your life.

13

Epilogue

I've been a family doctor for more than forty years, yet while I was researching this book I had to force myself to abandon many of my long-held beliefs about intellect and its eventual loss into the abyss of dementia. I had worried, too, that there wouldn't be enough that was positive and encouraging for the book to be useful to readers hoping to avoid or at least postpone dementia.

The first belief to be abandoned was that the brain was fully formed by adolescence, and that after early adulthood there was no possibility of further brain cell or intellectual growth. The accepted knowledge was that it was downhill all the way after the age of 25, with millions of neurones being lost and not replaced each year from then on.

Now we know that brain cells are constantly changing, renewing and making new and more connections with their neighbours and with similar cells further afield. Even in older ages, the brain can recover and regroup, and there must be ways in which we can enhance that process. The London cabbies' story was one of the first inklings of this. The story of the professional musicians strongly supported it. They showed that the more we use all five senses in co-ordination, the more connections our brain cells make and the more resistant they should be, in theory, to dementia.

This discovery is in tune with the next abandoned belief – that in normal life we use only a small part of the brain, and that the vast majority of our brain power lies unused. Ever more sophisticated brain-scanning systems now show that we use far more of our brains, even when completing simple tasks, than we thought just a decade or so ago. Many more areas of our brains 'light up' when we are asked to answer questions, solve problems, perform exercises and even when we sleep, than we knew about before we had the scans. The brain is a network of nerve pathways between cells that is far more complex, and has far more resilience and ability to heal and expand than we ever thought. In the near future we should know far more about how to manipulate these systems to avoid dementia, degeneration and losses of brain cells and pathways.

We are now learning something about how to do just that. The professional musicians have shown us part of this. I'm sure there are two aspects to their advantages over the rest of us. They have learned from an early age how to combine all five senses and to enhance their ability to co-ordinate their fine muscle actions with them. In doing so they have laid down many more pathways and connected many different parts of their brains in ways not seen in the rest of us.

But there is another aspect of a musician's life that differs markedly from the lives of the rest of us. It is essential for them to work closely with others, in orchestras and bands, and to be sociable beings, as well as being experts physically and mentally in their own fields. That gregariousness, I'm sure, is another way to keep all areas of their brains active, and hopefully more able to prevent dementia. Solitary pursuits, however intellectually challenging, such as writing, may not offer that same protection.

A third abandoned belief is that it's possible to 'train' one's brain by programmes, usually on-line, that purport to improve intellect. They just don't work. They may help you to be better at the task the 'trainer' has set, but not at anything else, and even that expertise doesn't last.

A fourth abandoned belief is that exercise has nothing to do with brain power, and that the slothful physically can still be alert mentally. All the studies show that physical exercise does seem to protect us against or postpone the onset of dementia. So get exercising. Maybe that's another benefit of being a professional musician – look at any orchestra and count those who are obese. They are as rare as those in my old school photograph. It is hard physical work producing music.

There is solid evidence – published in the prestigious *Proceedings of the National Academy of Sciences* in 2011 – to support the exercise theory. It comes from scientists at several US universities, who showed that if people aged 55 to 80 embarked on an exercise programme until they were walking briskly for 40 minutes three times a week, they not only improved their physical fitness, but increased the activity and size of the areas of the brain involved in memory. 'Control' adults of the same age who didn't walk showed the expected slight decline in the same areas. The study was too short and small to detect any difference in memory or intellect in the two groups, but the brain changes were real. It seems it is never too late to take up exercise or to improve your brain power.

A fifth abandoned belief is that there is some magic food that will protect or enhance our brain power. So many articles about dementia concentrate on trying to find a food that will help the brain. All the evidence is that supplements and extra vitamins and minerals over and above a normally varied diet don't help, and may even be counterproductive. Fish, meat, fruit (especially black soft fruits), vegetables and dairy products in good variety are the order of the day. Faddy diets are out.

I don't have to add absolutely no tobacco and very moderate alcohol consumption, but I've done so for completeness.

Best of all is that we can reduce our risk of dementia at any age in life. Our brains will respond. They don't die off bit by bit if we keep physically and mentally active – they do respond to a new approach. It's never too late to exercise, and to meet new friends and enjoy the company of old ones. And if you want to make a racket together, why not? Optimism is the key: keep it on you, and use it to open the locks in your brain.

The final belief to be abandoned is that as we age we become more depressed. The lie to that was given in 2010 when it was announced that the happiest time of most people's lives is around the age of 74. You don't have to let depression rule your old age. If you are down, get help. There is plenty around, from your medical team to your friends and the rest of your social circle. Enjoy life, and put the threat of dementia behind you.

Index